Living Every Day with Hope

*This is a book of daily reflections
by MA members for MA members*

Published by A New Leaf Publications, a department of
Marijuana Anonymous World Services
5551 Hollywood Blvd., #1043,
Hollywood, California 90028-6814 USA
+1.800.766.6779
www.marijuana-anonymous.org
A New Leaf Publications literature sales:
www.anewleafpublications.org

ISBN:

Living Every Day with Hope

*This is a book of daily reflections
by MA members for MA members*

Contents

Preamble

MARIJUANA ANONYMOUS is a fellowship of people who share our experience, strength, and hope with each other that we may solve our common problem and help others to recover from marijuana addiction.

The only requirement for membership is a desire to stop using marijuana. There are no dues or fees for membership. We are self-supporting through our own contributions. MA is not affiliated with any religious or secular institution or organization and has no opinion on any outside controversies or causes. Our primary purpose is to stay free of marijuana and to help the marijuana addict who still suffers achieve the same freedom. We can do this by practicing our suggested Twelve Steps of recovery and by being guided as a group by our Twelve Traditions.

- Life with Hope, third edition, page *xvii*

Preface

In 2007, an MA member longed for a book of daily reflections written by recovering marijuana addicts. They received a lot of hope and encouragement from daily readers of other fellowships, but wanted one that reflected their unique addiction. In a grassroots campaign, they started collecting original submissions at MA Conventions, Conferences, and home workshops. After several years, however, the load grew too heavy for a single person. Fifty-five submissions were turned over to World Services where progress idled for several years.

In 2019, a spiritual spark was reignited when a handful of MA members expressed interest in the advancement of the book. They picked up where others had left off and formed the MA Daily Reflections Subcommittee. They swiftly drafted a submission format, posted it to the website, and announced the demand at meetings. With the subsequent advent of virtual meetings, the appeal reached far and wide. Members, passionate about sharing their recovery, submitted reflections individually and at workshops. Like a wave, the number of submissions increased exponentially. Within just a couple of years, the subcommittee had enough submissions in hand. Finally, the reflections were assembled, refined, and approved for publication.

We express a tremendous gratitude to the array of recovering marijuana addicts who participated in the development of this 16-year labor of love. This book is a testament that together we can do what we could never do alone. We hope that reading it is as rewarding for you as it was for those who contributed, and that it proves valuable in your recovery journey.

Introduction

Living Every Day with Hope is a series of daily reflections written by marijuana addicts so readers might find inspiration in their recovery. There is a reflection for each day of the year, referencing a short quote from MA Conference–approved literature. All reflections were submitted by MA members between 2007 and 2021. With no minimum clean time requirement, all could participate. Each reflection ends with a final thought, such as a challenge for the day, a word of encouragement, or a simple concluding message.

The committee members made only minor edits in an effort to preserve the writer's original voice. Therefore, the reader will notice stylistic differences between reflections. As the label on a new tie-dye shirt describes each piece as one-of-a-kind, you will notice these reflections are just as unique. This book is organized in such a way that any day you read, you can receive a message of hope that sustains and strengthens your recovery. As you might hear in meetings, "take what you like and leave the rest."

January 1

Progress, not Perfection

"Step One: We admitted we were powerless over marijuana, that our lives had become unmanageable."

- *Life With Hope*, first edition, page 1

There was a crack deep within me, and once I accepted it—accepted that I am a marijuana addict—the light began to pour in. Taking each next right action, one day at a time, as long as I don't pick up, I am making progress. I don't have to do recovery or anything else with perfection. I have the freedom to make mistakes and learn and grow from them.

When in the depths of addiction to pot, my life was full of shame, fear, anxiety, worry, and paranoia. I tried so hard to overcome my addiction by myself—I expected that I should be able to. I tried to be perfect, and time and time again, I failed to meet my expectations. Each time I let myself down, I crashed deeper into my addiction, and a spiral of hopelessness and depression. Marijuana Anonymous has taught me that I do not have to do it by myself. I have the resources of my Higher Power, meetings, fellows and my sponsor to support me. I have the tools of our beautiful book, *Life with Hope*, the *MA Workbook*, and the Twelve Steps. By admitting my powerlessness over marijuana, and asking for help, I paved the way for peace, serenity, and inner transformation.

Ironically, by admitting my powerlessness, I began to have access to true spiritual power within me and beyond me. Where once my addiction was my biggest source of shame, I can now completely accept it and recognize that my addiction led me straight into a spiritual revolution, and a new way of living. The light found its way in through my broken and cracked old self.

Final thought: Just as a new year is born on this day, I too am renewed each and every day, one day at a time.

January 2

Honesty is Like Gravity

"Step One is about honesty, about giving up our delusions and coming to grips with reality. We had to look honestly at our relationship with marijuana and its effect on our lives."

- Life With Hope, first edition, page 1

Our fellowship starts with honesty. Honesty is like gravity. Once I can be truly honest with what using pot has done to my life, honesty will pull me out of my delusional state; it is the first step to returning me to sanity. The addict that lives inside wants to get me to use. The addict wants to convince me that marijuana is not a problem and that I need it to function.

I thought that I needed marijuana to be happy, to be sad, to go to sleep, to go to the movies, to go to dinner, to get on a plane, to be the first thing I did in the morning and to even wake up in the middle of the night to smoke it too. Honestly, I was trapped in a thick smoke of delusion. I had become a slave to marijuana and I almost lost everything just so I could smoke. I finally realized that losing everything just for that one thing (that joint) was truly insane!

Final thought: Today, I have decided to give up that one thing (marijuana) so I can have everything! It's honestly a sense of freedom that gets me higher than weed ever could.

January 3

Keep Coming Back

"Marijuana addiction differs...but internally, the same pain and anguish exist...An individual may wake up years into this chronic illness, without a reasonable understanding of how their life got so off track."

- A Doctor's Opinion about Marijuana Addiction, MA pamphlet

I had avoided using in high school because I was ambitious and wanted to get out of that tiny rural town. I had seen how pot had affected several of my friends and how they no longer wanted to participate in things like sports or musical events.

It still hurts to think how I turned my back on my family and made rare contact, usually to "borrow" money or make some excuse to avoid a holiday. It took two years to become totally addicted. When people who cared about me made comments on how I had changed, I truly thought they were fools for missing out on this glamorous decadence.

Things got scary more than once, but it wasn't until I went to a meeting and heard people sharing about "audio hallucinations" that I realized, though I claimed not to ever get paranoid on pot, other things had been happening. I kept going back to meetings and each time I could connect the dots a bit more about how pot had caused depression and hopelessness. I connected with people who had learned the hard way that this "soft" drug could steal your life and make the misery unbearable. I learned that cross addiction was real but I also learned about friendship and self-respect and a loving God, and for that I keep coming back.

Final thought: Today, I've gone from a long, slow decline to "happy, joyous, and free!"

January 4

Serenity and Acceptance

"...humility is the key to serenity and happiness."

- Life with Hope, first edition, page 34

"God, grant us the serenity..." I had no relationship to the word 'serenity' when I first came into recovery. It quickly became a core value in my life. I've learned to look at serenity as a practice, as a choice. Praying for serenity is an excellent alternative to smoking weed. I used to smoke because I was chasing after an experience of pleasure, of control, of centeredness. The more I smoked, the further away I felt from these experiences.

Being clean gives me the opportunity to truly live the life I want to live. When my body is being affected by the chemicals in marijuana, I actually have less control over my experience. When I am clean, and connected to the divine, I can choose my attitude, or ask for help from my Higher Power to direct me. Serenity means acceptance. Now, instead of smoking weed to try to feel better, I pray for serenity. It's actually much more effective. There's a saying, "clean and crazy" that describes a person who is not using substances but still has no serenity in life. To truly be clean, I pray for serenity. Serenity is sobriety. It is acceptance; it is prioritizing my connection to the divine over my character defects.

Final thought: Today, I will prioritize my serenity over all else. Nothing is more important than my connection to divine love.

January 5

Admitting Powerlessness Leads to Empowerment

"Many of us spent years trying to control our use of marijuana. We justified our using and rationalized that we could control it...All these efforts failed us."

- Life with Hope, first edition, page 1

I had to develop a relationship with my powerlessness over marijuana before I was ever ready to admit that I had a problem. It took me years of stepping into the ring with weed and getting hit harder and harder, knocked down over and over, before I came into the rooms and got honest about my addiction. I had a really hard time admitting my powerlessness because in the beginning weed worked for me—it was fun and then it became my medicine that I would look forward to every day. Finally, it became my greatest struggle and a symbol of my failure and broken heart.

Now, I have a relationship with honesty and recovery that empowers me each day to stay clean. I have an intimate relationship with powerlessness as a foundational spiritual principle upon which the rest of my recovery stands. I've been told that the only Step that one needs to work perfectly is Step One—admitting that I'm powerless over marijuana and that my life has become unmanageable.

Upon that spiritual foundation I build a profoundly powerful life in recovery, full of self-determination and service to others. It's one of the many paradoxes of my spiritual path—it's through admitting my powerlessness that I begin to gain real empowerment.

Final thought: Today, I will honestly admit my powerlessness over addictive behavior and upon that spiritual foundation, I will build an empowered life free of addiction.

January 6

The Twelve Questions

"Does your marijuana use let you live in a privately defined world?"

- The Twelve Questions, *Life with Hope,* third edition, page 192

The Twelve Questions really blew my mind the first time I heard them. I identify most with Question Seven. I loved getting high outside and going into the fantasy world. At first, I was really mad if my drug of choice was not available; how was I going to get to the fantasy?

Eventually, I was able to learn how to live in reality and, eventually, I was OK with it too. The main thing that helps me stay in reality is my Higher Power. I ask for help and listen for where to go and what to do; I wait for the direction and it always comes. The greatest thing about staying in reality is that there are other people there. I found that I really like working with others; one-on-one, volunteering for an event, or making 12-Step work possible. In these ways, I find joy in reality and the here and now.

Final thought: Today, I can be right where my feet are and I usually like it.

January 7

Me? A Derelict?

"A few of us were derelicts. In spite of all this, we still had difficulty admitting that we could no longer manage our own lives!"

- Life with Hope, second edition, page 3

The first few times I read Step One, I would see the term "derelict" and an image would pop into my mind of an unkempt, bearded vagrant, reeking of booze, cigarettes, and weed, eyes heavy from years of self-sabotage. I would confidently think "that wasn't me." One day though, I explored the definition of "derelict." Indeed, a person without belongings, or a home, or job, could be described as such, but "derelict" also describes something that has been neglected, misused, or left behind. Had I not done that to myself?

Years of marijuana use led me to neglect my soul, misuse my body (and lungs!), and leave behind goals and dreams that I was fully capable of achieving. I then realized that this seemingly far-fetched term actually defined my addiction!

Final thought: Today, I am no longer a derelict. I respect myself, my body, and my life—nourish it instead of neglect it, harness it instead of misuse it, and reclaim it instead of leaving it behind.

January 8

Denial to Honesty

"Until we admitted our powerlessness, denial kept us from realizing how unmanageable our lives had become. Our visions of achievement and our desires of being wise, loving, compassionate, or valued had remained mostly dreams. We rarely realized our potentials. We had settled for being merely functional."

- Life with Hope, first edition, page 3

The word "denial" is synonymous with being an addict. As an acronym (Denial - Didn't Even Notice I Am Lying), denial helps explain why I would promise not to use and then an hour later I would be smoking a joint. I wasn't even aware of the lies I was telling myself. I could lie to myself and believe it. Every lie that I believed took me farther from the life I wanted to live. I was living the fantasy of functionality.

One day I walked into the rooms of Marijuana Anonymous and was told that I needed to get honest with myself and my addiction. I had to take an honest look at my relationship with marijuana and the depths to which it had brought me. From that day onward it became easier to be honest with myself and with those in my life, and to face "life on life's terms."

Final thought: Today, I admit that I am powerless over marijuana, and by doing that, my life becomes more manageable!

January 9

Self-Acceptance

"We took a stride towards wisdom...we gained a tool, which we could use to take an objective look at ourselves. With the help and counsel of another person, we could confirm our findings. We used our human faculties, the counsel of another human being, and our relationship with a Higher Power to be born anew. This was the beginning of the experience of self-acceptance."

- Life with Hope, third edition, page 23

Before recovery, if you would have asked me if I was honest with myself, I would've said yes to you, but inwardly screamed no. I never really enjoyed looking at the dirty, grimy, unpleasant parts of myself. I thought I would implode if I had. I thought it would just be too painful. I'd have to own just how disappointed I was with those parts, how ashamed of them I was.

As I move into the new year and complete another chapter of my recovery, I can look at myself in the mirror with curiosity rather than disdain. I can acknowledge those parts that terrified me, rather than curse them. I can hug the little girl inside me and cry tears because instead of berating her for what she's done or felt, I'm accepting her in a way she hadn't known before. Through my recovery, I am learning to feel my wounds, listen to and be present for them, so that I can properly heal them. Through my recovery I'm tuning in. I'm becoming the person my Higher Power has always known I can be when I give myself the chance. I'm shedding. I'm renewing. I'm gently becoming what was always there for me to be and I'm so, so proud.

Final thought: Today, self-acceptance comes as I take a gentle look at what's there, and still love myself.

January 10

First Thought: Wrong

"The third stage of addiction is related to craving. The frontal cortex, where we think things through, plan things out, and alter our behavior to meet our own needs, is the primary part of the brain that is altered."

- *Life with Hope,* third edition, page *xxviii*

When I first stopped using marijuana, I was often assaulted by intense cravings to use again. Random thoughts of how and why I could use "one more time" came easily into my mind. As I stayed clean for a while, the intensity and frequency of cravings diminished; however, random thoughts of using did continue. Thoughts like these are not products of careful deliberation or executive brain functions. They are born out of the effects of marijuana withdrawal and out of old lifestyle habits.

It is important to dismiss such thoughts as products of my altered brain chemistry. The slogan "first thought: wrong" helps to remind me that my disease is responsible for cravings like these. I dismiss these thoughts without even analyzing why I'm having them; I just let them flow by. I am not accountable for an irrational first thought. I am accountable for my second thought and my first action.

Final thought: Today, I will let irrational first thoughts just flow by. I will remember "first thought: wrong."

January 11

The Principles

"Each step carries at least one main spiritual principle. We strive to apply these principles not only to the program and the fellows in it, but to all aspects of our lives."

- *MA Workbook*, first edition, 11th printing, page 57

When I am honest, I gain the trust I had lost.
When I have hope, I know that the future is bright.
My faith gives me the strength to stay sober.
To have courage allows me to do what I used to fear.
My integrity puts me in a state of wholeness.
Willingness guides me to the next right action.
By having humility I will face my defects.
Through reflection I can see what my life has become.
Practicing justice makes my world a better place to live.
With perseverance I can attain my goals.
Spiritual awareness keeps my Higher Power by my side.

Final thought: If I practice these principles today and every day I will be well on my way to living a life of joy while being a source of good in the world.

January 12

Higher Power

"As addicts... we forgot our mission; we forgot the other adventures that awaited us; we forgot about going home."

- The Story of the Lotus Eaters, Life with Hope, first edition, page xiv

God, grant me the serenity to accept the things

I cannot change (*people, places, and things*)

The courage to change the things I can (*myself*)

And the wisdom to know the difference (*your will for me*)

The First Step included admitting our lives were unmanageable. As an addict I have to try every day to release my desire to control. Every day is a practice of letting my Higher Power into my life. It's often easier to distinguish my Higher Power's will from my own after the fact. Every day is a practice of humility. Every day is progress if I allow it. Every day I remind myself to be gentle.

Final thought: Today, I will practice letting my Higher Power into my life. I will practice humility, and remind myself to be gentle.

January 13

Choose Your Pain

"Step One was the first step to freedom. We admitted our lack of power and our inability to control our lives. We began to acknowledge how mentally, emotionally, and spiritually bankrupt we had become. We became honest with ourselves. It was only by admitting our powerlessness in this first Step that we became willing to take the next eleven Steps."

- Life with Hope, third edition, page 5

The admission that Step One calls for will feel like a punch in the gut. My ego will fight to keep marijuana in my life because denial and resistance are its most potent fuels. It will be painful to concede to the fact that the control I thought I had over my life is an illusion. In truth, it is the arrogance of my ego that gave birth to and perpetuates the insidious cycle of addiction. Growth is never easy; it wouldn't be called "growing pains" otherwise; however, it is a well-known fact that nothing worthwhile ever comes easy. It is in the trials and tribulation that I discover there is strength in vulnerability.

Acceptance grants access to the power and wisdom of the universe; I need only practice stillness and faith to tap into the peace of being in the capable hands of my Higher Power. The cycle of addiction and the journey towards growth certainly comes with its own unique bundle of pain. I can either choose the pain of addiction or the pain of growth. The former leads to existential bankruptcy and the latter leads to the freedom and peace of an examined life. Addiction has been demanding the bankruptcy of my existence as payment for its promise of elusive euphoria. Growth will demand that I put in the work to earn the freedom and peace of an examined life. Pain is inevitable. Suffering is optional.

Final thought: Today, will you choose to chase the fantasy of euphoria or will you choose to earn your freedom?

January 14

Genuine Change

"It begins with a real desire to stop using, with a genuine change in our attitude, with a soul-transforming realization that we are finally willing to go to any lengths to change our lives."

- Life with Hope, first edition, page 4

This is my favorite line from *Life With Hope*. I just wanted to stop smoking. I just thought I could quit and move on with my life as it was. I thought I was a good person with a bad habit. I didn't realize that I was going to be changing my attitude. My attitude towards my addiction, and my connection to my family, friends and God were all going to go through an overhaul. The program and steps taught me how to change my life.

Final thought: Every day, I have a soul-transforming realization and for that I am grateful.

January 15

The Empowering Paradox of Admitting Powerlessness

"The entire foundation of our program depends on an honest admission of our powerlessness over addiction and the unmanageability of our lives. We are, however, responsible for our own recovery."

- Life with Hope, second edition, page 3

To me, being powerless over marijuana doesn't just mean that I cannot use in moderation, it also means that I have no control over the effect it has on me once it is in my body. No matter how much I wanted weed to help me feel connected or motivated, I increasingly felt isolated and lethargic. "Unmanageability" was hard to admit, as I had a life that looked outwardly functional and my bottoming-out was on a couch rather than in a gutter. At a meeting I heard, "Unmanageability is when your circumstances fall below your standards." My original standard was to live life to the fullest and use stories to change lives. In the end, I could hardly complete a thought, much less make eye contact. There had been a very gradual lowering of my standards as my circumstances descended into a haze.

Final thought: Only after accepting the things I cannot change in Step One, was I able to assume the responsibility of changing the things I can, through the following Steps and beyond.

January 16

Difficult Feelings

"Within the fellowship, we found that many of us had done the same kinds of things, had felt the same, and had experienced similar thoughts."

- *Life with Hope,* first edition, page 17

This too shall pass. Remember nobody's perfect. We are human beings and sometimes that has to be enough. It's not always the disease. In my addiction, I had no choice but to use marijuana when confronted with personal problems. In recovery, I get the opportunity to accept my humanity, to turn toward the pain rather than mask it with addictive substances and behaviors. Just for today, I will reach out and tell another addict about my personal problems, not for a fix, but to let them know what's going on. Our fellows often become our closest friends, and in this way we are doubly lucky.

Final thought: Carrying the message of recovery doesn't have to be going to a meeting or sponsoring somebody. It can be listening with a nonjudgmental ear, holding a space for the newcomer in our hearts, and giving back the gift that was so freely given to us.

January 17

Our Lives Had Become Unmanageable

"For some of us, Step One meant honesty for the very first time in our lives."

- Life with Hope, third edition, page 3

Over the years, I have come to a greater understanding of Step One. When I first came into the rooms, I admitted that I was powerless over marijuana, and my life had become unmanageable. How could I not see the wreckage of my life? It was a selfish way to look at my addiction and recovery, and it is not what Step One says.

What I have come to understand and accept is that, "We admitted we were powerless over marijuana." Not only was I powerless; my boss, my family and my partners were powerless over my marijuana addiction. It is not that they didn't care for me, it is that I made "our lives unmanageable," and they did not know how to deal with me. They left, abandoned, or fired me. It is not because I didn't care for them, it was because I was unable to care for them. I was caught in my own little drama of life. I was unable to see what they needed and wanted and I was unable to communicate with them in an honest and compassionate way.

By working these Steps and being of service to others, I had pulled my head out of the sand of denial and can now see that I can be a positive light in the lives of those around me.

Final thought: Today, I accept that my life is unmanageable and I ask my Higher Power to help all those in my life, including me, to be released from the burdens of this day.

January 18

Sponsorship is a Gift

"A relationship with a sponsor is an important tool in recovery. It is often the beginning of the development of an ability to trust others and communicate effectively."

- About Sponsorship, MA pamphlet

For me, having a sponsor is one of the greatest gifts of the program. It took me some weeks before I felt comfortable asking someone to work with me. I didn't feel worthy enough. I remember how uncomfortable I felt when I would end a phone call with my first sponsor and she would tell me she loved me. She was the first person in my life that I felt safe with, and I began to sow the seeds of learning how to trust another.

I came to the program not knowing how to trust. It was so wonderful to learn trust with this loving sponsor who I learned never judged me. She walked me through the first nine Steps, and then she moved away. Then I found another sponsor. I moved and found yet another wonderful person willing to help me work the Steps of this miraculous program. Letting someone know all my secrets, and know they still care for me, has been a transformative experience. It has helped me realize that I'm worthy of love, no matter what I've done or who I've been. Learning to trust that others care for me has helped me learn to care for myself.

Final thought: My sponsor is not a therapist, but another addict who helps me work the 12-Step program of recovery. I can't, but we can.

January 19

Spiritual Help

"In Step One we confronted our addiction, admitting that we were powerless over marijuana and that our lives had become unmanageable. We were then left with two alternatives: to stay as we were and continue using marijuana until we died, or to seek spiritual help."

- Life with Hope, second edition, page 5

What? Death or spiritual help? Those are our only alternatives? Surely, there must be other options. When I really thought about it, I had tried and exhausted every option besides spiritual help without success before coming to Marijuana Anonymous. In fact, before I came, I never even considered spiritual help to be an option.

After my first few MA meetings, I was glad to have help staying clean. I came to understand that help from any one or two of my fellows would not be enough and would lead me to disappointment or worse. Help that comes from within; that never leaves me if I seek it out. That help could possibly be enough for those times late at night, or when interaction with other people was not possible. I came to understand that spiritual help was often a quiet voice inside me that comforted and supported me. This voice told me that I did not need marijuana to make me whole, or normal, or fun. The more I listened to that quiet voice, the louder and stronger it became and the less I heard the voice inside me that lured me to use marijuana.

Final thought: For today, I embrace spiritual help as a constant loving companion.

January 20

Fantasy of Functionality

"We were living the fantasy of functionality."

- Life with Hope, second edition, page 2

While using marijuana, I believed that I had power and I was in control. I was able to do all of my daily tasks. I used marijuana, went to work, used marijuana, came home, used marijuana, cooked and cleaned, used marijuana, entertained company, and used marijuana. My life was great on the outside, but on the inside there was a nagging doubt. On my job, I couldn't possibly give 100 percent, with my friends I wasn't giving my all. I decided that I would stop smoking marijuana, but there was another lurking thought, "Why would you want to stop smoking, you have everything that you want?"

I was living the fantasy of functionality. I didn't have enough reasons to stop using marijuana until I tried to stop. That was when I realized that I truly had no power over using marijuana and I was not in control. Marijuana was a part of my functionality and I only looked like I had it all together when I did not. Quitting actually made my life look completely different. Instead of using before work, I prayed to my Higher Power, and was sent to a program called Marijuana Anonymous—my life had totally changed. Instead of using, I went to meetings.

Final thought: Today, my life has changed because my Higher Power sent me to the Marijuana Anonymous recovery program.

January 21

The Wisdom of Experience

"The guilty feelings born in our past start to fall away. We begin to feel a closeness and an intimacy with all of creation. In fact, the wreckage of our past actually starts to feel like a resource of experience from which we can begin to learn and grow."

- Life with Hope, third edition, page 23

Early in my sobriety I was overwhelmed with a sense of shame, guilt, and remorse over all the lost opportunities, errors in judgment, and bad decisions I'd made when I was using. I found inescapable the sense that my life had been a waste and that I had spent far too many years in active addiction. Certainly, there was truth underlying these feelings, but beyond grasping that truth, they did little to help me in my recovery, and potentially represented obstacles to my long-term sobriety and spiritual growth. I had to discover for myself that, "our experience can benefit others," even when, or especially when, it concerns mistakes I've made.

I felt a great sense of liberation from all those feelings of self-pity, remorse, and shame when I was able to share with others in the program the lessons gained from mistakes I'd made. Like everyone else, I was born without knowledge, understanding, or wisdom—all of which can be gained only in the struggle of one's own or another's struggle. If the suffering I endured as a result of my errors can save me and another from equal or worse suffering, then it was well worth it.

Final thought: Today, I have decided to leave self-pity, shame, and remorse behind in gratitude for the wisdom my experience offers me.

January 22

Letting Go of Everything

"...praying only for knowledge of God's will for us and the power to carry that out."

- *Life with Hope*, second edition, page 55

Lately, my sponsor keeps reminding me that I need to let go. I need to let go of my expectations, my wants, and learn to accept what is. Letting go is another way of surrendering. An important lesson I've learned in recovery is that I don't have to do this perfectly. In recovery a more gentle approach is progress, not perfection. Recently, I heard a new saying, "my progress is perfect."

I've discovered that no matter what spiritual truths I learn in recovery, I need to relearn them over and over again. This is what keeps me coming back to meetings, no matter what. I have an amazing forgetter, and I need the messages I hear in meetings to remind me of spiritual truths that keep me clean.

"Let go and let God," was the first slogan that I grabbed onto in early recovery. I would say it over and over in my head while trying to learn how to meditate. Mostly I think about letting go, but I often forget about letting God. When I remember to let my Higher Power row the boat, I have the opportunity to be happy, joyous, and free.

Final thought: Remembering the 11th Step, I pray to know my Higher Power's will for me, AND the power to carry out that will. Then, I let go of the rest.

January 23

The Depth of Addiction and Recovery

"The only requirement is a desire to stop using marijuana."

- Preamble, *Life with Hope*, first edition, page *xi*

One of my character defects is that I can be quite judgmental. When I was getting high, I thought everyone should live like I did. I thought I was just smart at finding the key to living a hedonistic, selfish life. When I got clean, I would judge people who introduced themselves as addicts. Didn't they know how to pick their poison, their "drug of choice?"

I was glad when the dangers of cross addiction sunk in. I finally realized that my years of "white knuckle abstinence" as a solution was an illusion. Years had been added to my suffering—and my loved ones' pain—because I dragged out my lack of surrender for so long. I have a tendency toward behavior that reflects a bone-deep addiction. I get addicted to substances and attitudes, feelings, and opinions.

Thank God, I have other addicts to talk to, so that I can recognize when this type of obsessive behavior comes up. We get honest, we share our experience, strength, and hope. We get a good laugh and sometimes a good cry. We get real and get a life beyond our wildest dreams.

Final thought: Today, I have freedom from my addictive behavior, self-talk, and attitudes.

January 24

Keeping It Simple

"Our program is not easy, but it is simple."

- How it Works, *Life with Hope*, third edition, page 193

I have a tendency to make things more complicated than they have to be. I like complicated. I find it interesting, and exciting, and it keeps my overactive brain entertained. When I came to MA meetings, and we read "How it Works," I heard the above quote over and over. Eventually, after a few months, the words started to sink in. Apparently, if I wanted to stay clean from marijuana, I would have to keep it simple. I didn't like this, but I knew what I'd been doing the whole time when I was using wasn't working for me. I needed to be willing to try something new. I tried to remember to keep things simple.

Talk about not easy; it was hard for someone who had been overcomplicating things her whole life to try to simplify life! I started avoiding disagreements with people. If someone had a different opinion, I didn't bother to state mine if they didn't ask. I just let it go. I knew I needed to prioritize self-care, so I made it a priority to eat and exercise and bathe each day. It was boring, and I still bristle against simplicity. Every time I see myself adding new complications into my life, I ask my Higher Power to help me be willing to keep it simple.

Final thought: Today, I will ask my Higher Power to help me to keep things simple so that I have room in my life to do the hard work of recovering.

January 25

Self-Forgiveness

"Recovery does not happen all at once. It is a process, not an event."

- *Life with Hope,* third edition, page 5

Recovery means a daily reprieve from the insanity and emotional unmanageability of active addiction. It is based on my spiritual condition in this moment. I can go anywhere and face any trigger if I am in a fit spiritual condition. On the other hand, if my spiritual condition is weak, I can relapse without being exposed to any triggers. Step One promises I will relapse if I do not continue to maintain a spiritual program. If I am not moving forward in my recovery and step work, then I am moving backward toward relapse. There is no such thing as staying still in the process of recovery. Reading this daily reflection book moves me forward each day, away from the negative consequences of marijuana use.

All that occurs in life is simply part of the process. I can choose to label it good or bad. Speaking with my fellows helps me to see the only thing that really matters: the next right step. If I can just focus on doing the next right thing in front of me, then the path forward will unravel in front of me. If I veer off this path, it can become hard to see the next right thing to do. In that case, I will simply practice self-forgiveness. Through self-forgiveness, the fog of guilt and shame is lifted. I can see the next right step in front of me.

Final thought: Today, I will continue to walk the path of recovery and accept my duty to do the next right thing in front of me.

January 26

A New Way of Living

"Our complete surrender and a new way of life were essential to our recovery."

- Life with Hope, second edition, page 4

I remember feeling so fearful when I faced the task of actually quitting pot. What would happen? It felt like I was stepping into the abyss. Would I be cradled by some invisible force? How will I be able to sleep? By the time I finally quit for good, after years of relapse after relapse, I had faced these fears over and over. On my own, I had lasted for maybe 30 days until I smashed head-on into feelings with which I couldn't sit. My marriage and career were at risk, and my emotional state was teetering on collapse.

Since arriving in MA, I have been supported and included by my loving fellows and am never alone. They loved me until I was able to love myself. By admitting that my addiction was out of control, I gained the confidence to surrender my will to my understanding of a loving God. When I was plagued by recurring internal false narratives, I learned how to slow down the mental onslaught and turn down the volume. I realized that my guilty obsession over my perceived failed potential was merely self-imposed emotional blackmail. I started letting go of my long-held system of self-sabotage.

In MA, I learned a new language and began a new way of living. In a short amount of time I felt relief, and the urge to use pot was lifted. I began to do service and stayed with it. I find that I receive more in return than I give, which is a reason to continue to serve.

Final thought: Today, I will watch and listen for God's will for me.

January 27

Higher Power's Guidance

"We need to keep in mind that we pray only for knowledge of God's will for us and the power to carry that out."

- Life with Hope, second edition, page 57

Before I got clean, worrying was a full-time job. I thought that if I worried about something, it wouldn't happen. It was a bit shocking when I heard the phrase, "worrying is praying for something bad to happen." I've learned that whatever I focus on increases. Practicing Step Eleven helps me remember to put my focus where it belongs, on my Higher Power. For years in recovery, I would pray to be shown my Higher Power's will, but neglected to ask for the power to carry it out.

Today, I try to remember the entire wording of Step Eleven, "Sought through prayer and meditation to improve our conscious contact with God, as we understood God, praying only for knowledge of God's will for us and the power to carry that out." As I pray, I enter the spirit of the world and remember that I am connected to everything. I pray for joy and gratitude. I ask to be shown what I need to do and say this day. I start each day thanking my Higher Power for my recovery, and ask to stay clean this day.

Final thought: May I turn to my Higher Power when unsure, and ask for guidance as well as the power to carry it out.

January 28

Meditation Works

"It has been said that prayer is talking to God and meditation is listening to God."

- Life with Hope, third edition, page 54

I tried to meditate 25 years ago on the dirty carpet of a church basement next to a noisy breathing fellow. I operated for the next 25 years believing that meditation was not for me. After a six year relapse that brought me to the depths of isolation from others—and especially God—I threw myself into my program of recovery, willing to do anything my sponsor suggested.

I am so grateful to have come to meditation again. I started by attending the amazing meditation meetings in my district. I found that when I focused on my breathing and let my thoughts come and go without fixating on them, a quietness or stillness came to me. I had tried to achieve this state by using marijuana, but it never quite worked. I avail myself of guided meditations online, some are as brief as three minutes. Gradually I am learning to find that state without these tools, but I am so grateful to have the help.

Now, as a daily practice and particularly in times of stress, I have access to quieting my mind, releasing anxiety, and listening for my right path. Marijuana slowed me down mentally, but it didn't ease the incessant chatter and doubt that blocked me from my Higher Power. Finding the still, small voice that has always been there for me helps me be more compassionate to myself and others as we walk through this life.

Final thought: Today, I cultivate more loving relationships by sitting in stillness with my Higher Power.

January 29

At Peace with Myself

"Many of us spent years trying to control our use of marijuana."

- *Life with Hope,* third edition, page 3

For years, I struggled with weed, which means that I struggled with myself. Reading the examples in the *Life with Hope* book in Step One brought back all the times I fought with myself. I made rules I would break, hid weed in places I would find, and gave it to friends I would call. I made promises I knew I couldn't keep. Every day, I was struggling with either smoking or not smoking. When I stopped smoking, I stopped the struggle. There is no more fighting because there is nothing to fight about. I no longer let weed get in the way of my being honest—a person of integrity who is integral, whole, and undivided.

Final thought: Today, I live in peace with myself.

January 30

Gratitude and Acceptance

"I am grateful to the many people over the years who have participated and are participating in my recovery. I always had a life. Thanks to Marijuana Anonymous, I now have a life worth living."

- A Life Worth Living, Life with Hope, second edition, pages 167-168

I once read that gratitude and acceptance are the two most important tools in recovery. I have found this to be true for me. When I'm in acceptance, I cease fighting what I cannot change. When I remember gratitude, I realize I have many blessings to be grateful for, starting with my sobriety and recovery.

At five years clean and sober I went through a very traumatic event. Early in my recovery, I would hear at meetings that, "God never gives you more than you can handle." For a while, I found this comforting. After this traumatic event, I felt so overwhelmed and unable to cope, that I got mad at my Higher Power for giving me much more than I could handle. After a lot of recovery work, I changed that phrase to, "life sometimes gives you more than you can handle, that's why you need a Higher Power."

As I crawled back from that, I also realized that my addiction focuses on the negative. It is always focused on what's wrong. To change this negative focus, I began to practice gratitude. For the first seven years of my recovery, gratitude was an annoying topic at a meeting, especially in November. Now, gratitude is a daily practice that helps my recovery. Today, I believe that acceptance really is the key to serenity. Fighting what is happening in my life never helps. When I accept life as it is, the next right thing becomes clear.

Final thought: Today, I give thanks for the blessings in my life, starting with my clean and sober life, and my recovery.

January 31

Freedom from Fear

"We have found that freedom from fear is much more important than freedom from want."

- *Life with Hope,* second edition, page 68

I used to think I had control over my life, or at least I had convinced myself that I was in control because it kept my fears somewhat at bay, though I now know that was denial and delusion. It wasn't until I found my mental health spiraling completely out of control, using the most marijuana I had ever used before and finally reaching my bottom, that I had to take a hard look at myself.

After finding MA, I was asked to be honest and deal with my fears head-on. With baby steps at first, I learned to be courageous despite feeling vulnerable while sharing the imperfect parts of myself in meetings. I remember the monumental effort it took to sit down for my Fourth Step inventory and I remember the ensuing panic attack, triggered by overwhelming shame, fear, and resistance. After a good long cry, I reached out to another fellow who helped me put words to the experience I had just had.

While in active addiction, I had been in survival mode, so I hadn't had the luxury of feeling my fears. It's only now that I'm gaining access to a sense of security, that I can have the emotional and spiritual space to feel and face my fears with the unwavering love of my Higher Power, the wisdom of the Twelve Steps to guide me, the support of this beautiful fellowship, and a growing practice of self-compassion.

Final thought: Today, I will acknowledge my fear and hold space for it, but I will choose to draw on my hopes, my strength, and my connection to my Higher Power to vanquish that fear. "We take these steps for ourselves, not by ourselves."

February 1

I Grew Through Step Two

"It is not necessary to say yes. It is, however, important to stop saying no. Observe the reality around you and the recovery taking place within MA. One only has to stop fighting."

- Life with Hope, third edition, page 8

I had said no, no, no, powerless? Not me,

But in reading those Twelve Questions...an addict I must be...

This label, this admission, filled me with shame and dread,

But my sick thinking and doing, it nearly left me dead.

When I put down the vape pen, I saw I had another problem instead,

With nothing else external to blame, I surrendered—it was my head!

Paranoid, closed-off, skeptical, no "G-o-d" for me, thanks,

So resistant to help 'til I learned...it's my perception, it "stanks!"

So maybe I'll put one toe over the line,

Instead of a fervent no, I said OK, maybe? Fine?

Though no concrete proof of a Being more powerful than me,

There was recovery happening, that much I could clearly see.

Perhaps I'll never fully understand this divine universal loving being,

But I'm grateful my journey to sanity is at long last beginning!

Final thought: Today, I will open my eyes to reality and see the beautiful and inspiring recovery journeys unfolding around me in MA.

February 2

Healing of the Spirit

"We practice spiritual principles, not religion."

- Life with Hope, first edition, page 9

The ability to practice the spiritual principles of my program does not depend solely on any religious beliefs rooted in the acceptance of an all-knowing, all powerful deity. The path to a spiritual awakening can also be found in the healing and growth of my "Inner-Spirit" by living in a "Good Orderly Direction." I came into recovery suffering from low self-esteem and self-loathing. Not only had my addiction to marijuana isolated me from society, but it also isolated me from a thoughtful awareness of my own individual identity, self-worth, and values. I had no ability to accept or forgive my own human frailties. My addiction to marijuana only fed the negative conceptions I had of myself as being a worthless failure. My spirits were sputtering flames which cast no warmth or light on anything around me.

By practicing the spiritual principles of the program, I learned to treat myself and others with kindness, fairness, acceptance, tolerance, and love. Like a cheerleader at a spirit rally who stands before the crowd seemingly confident, happy, and enthusiastic about their own lives and abilities, a spiritually healthy person leads by example, demonstrating to others through their daily actions and interactions, that they have gained a positive conception of themselves as functioning, productive, self-aware members of the fellowship and society. I have become a person who does not think less of myself, but thinks of myself less.

Final thought: Today, let me practice healing my Inner Spirit by recognizing in myself and others our common humanity, value, and inherent self-worth.

February 3

I Am Learning

"...recovery from addiction requires resources beyond the capacities of any one individual addict."

- Life with Hope, first edition, page 8

I get it. I am a marijuana addict. I know that I did not want to be one. I thought that the subtle smoky ally of mine was my friend. It was for a long time. Through most of my twenties I could bounce back the next day and hit the reset button and not suffer any consequences. I didn't realize my short temper, my dirty laundry, the undone dishes, the girlfriend that cried; I didn't realize these were signals! I am clean today. My ego is too big and I think I know everything; still my sponsor loves me like a brother, like a friend who can handle the insanity of someone who desperately wants to stay clean.

I am seventy-five days clean at midnight. My bed is made. I ate a salad today, a salad with kale! What is going on: I pray, I remain malleable, and most of all, I am grateful. I am so grateful. The smoky demon is all around me and somehow I am protected.

Final thought: Today, I am grateful that I was willing to go to any lengths to change my life. Teach me more.

February 4

Came to Believe

"Our insanity was evident as we repeated the same behavior over and over, and somehow expected different results."

- Life with Hope, first edition, page 5

Admitting my powerlessness and unmanageability is a challenge that will take time. I need not be defined by my suffering and desperation. By listening to others' stories I learned that my experience is, in fact, not unique, but shared by many. Slippery self-deception and self-disgust does not serve me. By becoming a part of a group that loves and supports me, I am given tools to combat loneliness and I'm drawn out of my isolation. As I put together periods of clean time, my internal dialogue is calmed and the chaos is reduced. There is another way to live.

Insanity sometimes is just being "out of order." I took rewards before actually earning them. I fed addiction at the expense of my peace of mind. In recovery, I learn to reach out to others and find help. I engage in a new way of life that offers hope. As I become open to re-ordering my priorities and place trust in the acceptance and wisdom of a loving Higher Power, my crazy-making cycles are diminished. When I loosen my vice-grip on the levers of my addiction, faith becomes within reach. I am not alone.

Final thought: Today, I will be sensitive to signs of a Higher Power in and around me.

February 5

Come As You Are

"There is room in MA for all beliefs, or none...We all have a place here. There is no conflict. For each of us, a power greater than ourselves...can be any positive, powerful thing that we are comfortable with."

- Life with Hope, first edition, page 9

If this is a disease of self-loathing, then thank God for Step Two. I don't think it even matters what you call your Higher Power. I just know that my Higher Power must be ever-loving, ever-accepting, ever-cheering me on, so that I cannot help but begin to like myself as a result of working these Steps.

When I put down the weed, a relationship to a Higher Power actually becomes possible. I'm not sure what it was that I thought I found before because I sure kept smoking for those spiritual effects! I've learned there are just some brains that cannot handle a mind or mood altering substance without devastating effects and consequences. I had one of those brains; yet another reason to hate myself. I have learned by the gentleness of my Higher Power that there is simply no room to hate myself for anything. I began to trust in my ability to face life without the help of marijuana's filter. What I found is that it's not that bad, that I am lovable, and that every little thing is going to be alright.

Final thought: Today, I will let go of being right about myself being all wrong and surrender to that force of love.

February 6

Action Without Agenda

"We take action and leave the results of our request to our Higher Power."

- Life with Hope, first edition, page 34

Throughout my using career, I put off important decisions until some future date when conditions were right. What those perfect conditions were, I never really got around to figuring out, but I felt that now was not the right time. Why didn't I take action in the past? Was it fear? Was it because I was too stoned to get off the couch? It possibly had to do with the fact I never really learned the skills to make my dreams a reality.

In recovery, I learn that the present moment is all I really have. Now is the perfect time for action. I know I am supported by a universe of endless possibilities, a strong fellowship in Marijuana Anonymous, and a loving Higher Power. Action is my driving motivation, not the results that follow.

Final thought: Today, I approach life with clear intent, but no set agenda. I know my Higher Power is always looking after me.

February 7

Tools of Recovery

"Do you smoke marijuana to avoid dealing with your problems?"

- The Twelve Questions of Marijuana Anonymous, *Life with Hope*, second edition, page xvii

One of the most beneficial lessons I've learned in recovery is how to deal with problems. When any difficulty came my way I depended on pot to help me solve the problem. It never did. I remained under the illusion that somehow marijuana could do what I couldn't do for myself. I became a victim. I had no other resources. Over time I believed that the solution to all my troubles, big or small, was dope. I think I even looked for difficulties so that I could get high. Life itself became my problem and marijuana my only solution. I'm reminded of the expression, "when all you have is a hammer, everything becomes a nail." Pot became my useless hammer. I used it to try to fix everything that came along. I had no other resources.

Now in recovery, I have new and better tools. In this program I use meetings, a sponsor, the Steps, and most of all, a belief in a Higher Power to help me deal with all that life has to offer.

Final thought: In recovery, I find a clear path to a more rewarding and fulfilling life.

February 8

Courage to Look at Ourselves Honestly

"In the instant that we faced our fears, we began to overcome them."

- Life with Hope, first edition, page 19

Coming into the recovery process, I felt burdened by a seemingly unshakable sense of shame. I could no longer turn to marijuana for anesthetization and without the haze of marijuana, I had to face the wreckage that my prior actions/inactions had caused. I was flooded with memories of how I had put my addiction above all else. I had squandered my education, stolen money from friends, and engaged in dangerous situations in order to score. I married a fellow drug addict to ensure that my marijuana use would never be challenged, and I cheated on him without a second thought when he restricted my supply. How could I have fallen so far from my values? I had lost my integrity and the thought of making a searching and fearless moral inventory felt daunting.

Fortunately, not one of us must face this challenge alone. Through ongoing commitment to working with my sponsor, I was able to face these fears and dig into my past with support; I can lance fear and shame in order to find healing. "We are only as sick as our secrets." Today I can look at my character defects as challenges—opportunities for furthering my spiritual evolution and movement towards my authentic self. No one is perfect—the only thing I must do is be aware of my words and actions thereby keeping "my side of the street clean."

Final thought: Today, I give myself grace. Our Higher Power is always with us, waiting for us to be ready for 'relief from these burdens of self.'

February 9

Opportunities for Growth

"We did whatever we could to make other people, places, and things be what we wanted. Since this proved to be impossible, we would be hurt and blame others for our problems. So we tried even harder to control and consequently suffered even more."

- Life with Hope, first edition, page 11

It used to really annoy me when I heard people in meetings say, "I'm grateful to be an addict." All I could see from being an addict were problems: fear, shame, guilt, and depression—not to mention the legal problems, lost jobs, failed relationships, and poor health. After a while I began to realize it was those problems, and the desperation they caused, that brought me to Marijuana Anonymous.

It was in MA where I was finding a whole new way of life. I began to see how my problems really were the "price of admission" to a spiritual life. As I continue to learn and grow in the program, I begin to see that a "problem" is really a solution trying to find me. When a part of my life isn't working, the Steps and the program give me a chance to look squarely at that situation and ask myself, "How can I learn and grow from this?" It's a wonderful ability that I learned in the rooms of MA and through working the Steps.

Today, I am not dominated by "problems," even when parts of my life aren't working. There are a lot less of those now that I'm clean. More importantly my eyes have been opened to a new way of seeing things: one where everything really is part of the path I have chosen to walk and for that I am truly grateful.

Final thought: Today, I will ask my Higher Power to help me see my "problems" as opportunities for learning and growth.

February 10

The Emotional Roller-Coaster

"One of the joys of being clean is the return of the full range of human emotions."

- Life with Hope, first edition, page 35

As a marijuana addict, I have experienced mood swings. Incredible joy and happiness can quickly move to utter despair in a matter of moments. Sometimes these quick changes in my emotions can be very confusing. As I gain time in recovery, I spend more time in the world of affairs, spreading my wings, and experiencing life to the fullest. These experiences will no doubt come with the fullness of the human condition; this means there will be experiences that will make me happy and those that will make me incredibly sad.

Also, there are some experiences where I will have to wait and see what happens; sometimes these are the hardest to bear. Today, I will embrace my feelings—good, bad, or indifferent. I know that these feelings are a gift from my Higher Power as proof positive that I am fully engaged in life, and truly living life on life's terms.

Final thought: Today, I embrace my emotions. I know that my Higher Power is working in my life today.

February 11

From Loneliness to Hope

"Some of us believe in no deity; a Higher Power may be the strength gained from being a part of, and caring for, a community of others."

- Life with Hope, first edition, page 7

Growing up as an only child, in a family ruled by addiction, I spent years feeling alone and afraid. In college, I started using marijuana and it eased an anxiety so deeply embedded inside of me, I hadn't even realized it was there. Eventually, though, the weed stopped working, and my addiction reached the point where it told me I would die of those feelings if I didn't use.

By the time I reached MA, I was terrified of that addict voice inside my head. I didn't trust myself to stay clean on my own. The only place I felt truly safe and free from cravings was while I was sitting in a Marijuana Anonymous meeting. I cried out to God to rescue me so many times as a child, and got no response. Could I risk such a huge disappointment again?

Now I realize that God, as I understand God, was already working in my life. It was in those rooms and meetings that held me, and kept me safe in early recovery. Since then, I've walked through multiple spiritual "deserts"—times when I felt that utter loneliness and disconnection from a power greater than myself. I know that those feelings may return in the future. The difference now is, I know I need never remain lonely and afraid, because I can always find love and connection in a meeting of Marijuana Anonymous.

Final thought: May I remember that God, as I understand God, can always be found in the care I can feel for others, and the care they can feel for me.

February 12

Came to Believe

"Some of us were just too smart for our own good. We thought we had it all figured out. We felt intellectually superior. 'I can do anything I set out to do....Knowledge is power!' Yet we were faced with the paradox of our own addiction. Our best thinking brought us to our bottom. What we learned is that recovery from addiction requires resources beyond the capacities of any one individual addict."

- Life with Hope, second edition, page 8

I found myself putting off anything I set to do until tomorrow. Just use once more and then I'll do it. This lasted for years. Years of saying, "I'll get to it tomorrow," as marijuana kept its grip on me. Even after cobbling together some time, I thought that I must be able to use safely now. In short time, I found myself back in the miserable isolation of my active addiction, and with every relapse, it got worse and worse.

The disease of addiction is delusional, it tricks me into thinking I don't have an addiction. It's also progressive, because the depravity of my actions with each relapse grew and grew. My disease, as it is often said, was doing push-ups, while I worked the Steps and took service commitments.

I don't know what this power greater than myself is, but that doesn't matter to me today. It is not me; it is a power that I see in the courage and grace of my fellows. It is the power that I see in natural events. It changes, and that's OK. I cannot do this on my own. Recovery from addiction requires resources beyond me. I came to believe that a power greater than myself could restore me to sanity, and I stopped obsessing over what that power is.

Final thought: Today, I believe that a power greater than myself can restore me to sanity, and I don't need to know exactly what that power is for it to do so.

February 13

Letting Go of Egotistical Thinking

"Step Two: *Came to believe that a Power greater than ourselves could restore us to sanity.*"

- *Life with Hope,* first edition, page 5

I first heard, "I'm an egomaniac with an inferiority complex," at an MA meeting. I can relate to this statement. I seem to be on both sides of a spectrum of self-esteem. At times I think of myself as some great knowledgeable person that others look up to, and at other times I think of myself as a worthless loser. I have learned through this program that my self-centered thinking is at the core of this dichotomy. During my life I felt responsible for much of what was going on outside of myself and developed a belief that I could control it.

In recovery I have been learning that I am responsible for my actions and God is responsible for the results. I must focus on the right action for me and not let fear or desire for results affect that focus. I am trying to learn humility, to let go of my self-centered egotistical thinking. My bad habit of judging people, including myself, has diminished as I work the program. I am slowly learning to accept myself, others, and life, as is, instead of expecting them to be something I have conceived.

Life continues to turn out so much differently than my ideas and plans of how I wanted it to be, and this is very painful at times. I am, however, experiencing levels of joy and fulfillment that I could never have dreamt of, and it is clear now that God knows what is best for me and my loved ones. Today, I like myself most of the time. I still do experience periods of self-hatred and inflated ego, but they are less frequent now and the duration is shorter.

Final thought: Higher Power is saving me from the bondage of self, and I am grateful.

February 14

God, As We Understand God

"If we have negative associations with the terms 'God' or 'Higher Power,' we are free to use whatever word or words are acceptable to us."

- Life with Hope, second edition, page 56

For years in recovery, I struggled with the concept of "God" or "Higher Power" because I could never conceive of God as a loving father/mother/friend. God, as I understood God, was all-encompassing; in each and every one of us and in all things, living and inanimate. God was in every emotion, instinct and passion—in love, justice and morality. How could I think of God as someone I could talk to? It was not until I could accept the limitations and imperfection of language to describe my understanding of God, and to accept that language is all I have to describe it.

I could use the words God or Higher Power as a convenient shorthand and smile at its oversimplification. Although it took me many years, once I stopped getting tripped up on the words God or Higher Power, I was finally able to use prayer and meditation to establish a conscious contact with God as I understand God.

Final thought: For today, I will not allow life's imperfections to keep me from obtaining all of the gifts this program has to offer.

February 15

Awakening

"Our new attitudes bring about self-esteem, inner strength, and serenity that is not easily shaken by any of life's hard times."

-Our Awakening, *Life with Hope,* third edition, page 61

For me the Awakening resonates. I feel I am A-waking up! I am in recovery and the cobwebs are clearing. I am beginning to move about in the world more mindfully with the help of Marijuana Anonymous. When I was smoking, when life got "lifey" I reacted, usually making things worse; I whipped things up! I was impatient, and felt "poor me."

Listening to fellows in MA meetings, I hear that life is complicated for all people. All people have stresses in their lives. I am not alone. Regardless of what is happening around me, (I now try to say AROUND me vs. TO me) I am learning to NOT overreact and realize I can be unflappable. I breathe and remember to let go and let God. When I can do that, I feel peaceful and A-wake.

Final thought: Today, with God's help, please help me learn to be a mountain in any storm.

February 16

Step Two

"We began to see the possibility that our beliefs about ourselves, formed while using, had been mistaken. We saw that our perceptions had been based in delusion."

- *Life with Hope*, first edition, page 6

I started smoking pot because I was uncomfortable and unhappy, and I kept on doing it long after it started making me feel worse, not better. I thought that unhappiness was my lot in life. I thought I was doing life wrong; didn't have what it took to be happy, successful, and loved and that my life just was not going to work out.

I came to Marijuana Anonymous thinking I just needed to quit smoking and everything would be fine. Because I stuck around, got involved, got honest, took the suggestions, and most of all, worked the Steps, I was able to accept myself as I am. I am a person with a disease, doing the best I can with what I have. I also got a new goal, not the "happiness" of ego gratification and getting what I want, but the peace, serenity, and freedom of living life on life's terms, one day at a time. Most of all, I learned that I am OK, and I am loved. I belong in the human race just as I am, and it is actually possible for me to be happy, joyous, and free.

Final thought: Today, I know that peace and serenity are available to me, so long as I stay clean and keep practicing these principles in all my affairs.

February 17

Everyday Miracles

"Observe the reality around you and the recovery taking place within MA. One only has to stop fighting."

- *Life with Hope,* second edition, page 7

Too often, I find myself demanding a "lightning bolt occurrence" to tell me that I am on the right path. Yet when I am able to pause and look around me, I often start to see how connected every strand of my life actually is. While it is easy to attribute events to happenstance and serendipity, it takes humility on my part to acknowledge the gifts that my life presents me with on a daily basis. Chance and luck are most certainly a part of my life—but I can't lose sight of the fact that both are part of a bigger picture that I can't see.

Final thought: Today, I can choose to see life as a series of random coincidences, or for the miracle that it really is.

February 18

Emotional Sobriety

"Addiction is a terminal disease that does not go into remission simply because we're not using. Constant vigilance is critical if we are to keep this disease at bay."

- Life with Hope, first edition, page 68

It is important for me to remember that I can't do recovery alone. I need MA meetings and the fellowship of other recovering addicts. Other addicts understand the pain that I have felt when using, and the joy that I feel now. My sponsor is someone who listens and offers advice when I need it. Growth opportunities come my way and I can work the Twelve Steps again.

My Higher Power has given me the gift of recovery. My Higher Power is always there for me. I can pray to do my Higher Power's will and listen when I meditate. I am someone who loves to give, and help others, and I can do this by being of service. I can be of service by attending a meeting or by being involved in a MA World Service Conference. I can give a message of hope by sharing my story of recovery. I am grateful that I can help the addict who still suffers. I am grateful to those who came before me and offered their loving help. I am grateful that I have been transformed from an addict full of sorrow into someone who is truly "happy, joyous, and free" every day.

Final thought: Today, I know that I can meet life's challenges of pain, fear, and hopelessness with love, peace, and serenity.

February 19

The Care of a Higher Power

"It was a thrilling experience to start a relationship with a Higher Power that I felt cared for me."

- A Slave to Marijuana, Life with Hope, third edition, page 102

I was raised in a religious environment. I lost my connection to the notion of a paternal, omnipresent, judgmental God-in-the-sky while I was in my teens. Coming into the rooms of Marijuana Anonymous I was confronted with the need and desire to develop a new relationship with a Higher Power that resonated with me.

At first, I was drawn to the God of my youth through habit but, as time passed, my connection with my God has deepened, shifted, and transformed into male, female, genderless, strict, flexible, micromanaging, hands-off. I have tried on the feeling of my God.

Now I have a friend, ally, and loving partner in my Higher Power. I converse with my HP, I laugh with my HP, I yell at my HP and I am humbled and grateful to be guided and cared for by my Higher Power. I am loved, and I am loving, and living through the will of my God.

Final thought: Today, I allow myself to be cared for and to care through the will of my Higher Power.

February 20

Focus On What's Yours, Only

"We saw that a power greater than ourselves was doing for us what we could never do alone."

- *Life with Hope,* first edition, page 9

Step Two tells me to remember that I am not God. I do not control other people or things. With the help of my Higher Power, I can control my behavior. In order to control my behavior, I must make choices. The choice to not smoke pot today can only come from a focused mind, a mind that is clear about what is in my control and what is not. When I try to own issues and problems that are not mine to own, I will set myself on the path to disappointment which can lead to frustration, disillusionment, and self loathing. This is a perfect recipe for relapse.

Final thought: Today, I choose to focus on the things I can control.

February 21

Sharing is Service

"We cannot keep the gifts the program has given us unless we give them away to others. We share our experiences and learn from each other. None of us can survive, and the fellowship cannot endure, unless we carry the message of recovery. We have found that those who keep coming back to the fellowship have a better chance of staying clean and sober."

- Life with Hope, second edition, pages 73-74

Giving back to others by being of service, sponsoring, and sharing experience, strength, and hope have been the crucial pieces that complete the puzzle of long-term sobriety. I have found that my chances of staying clean have increased ten-fold when I made the decision to give back to others within the program.

The thought of relapsing did not cross my mind the moment I picked up my first service commitment. Relapse was a part of my journey (as I have relapsed a handful of times), but since I began serving my fellows, I haven't relapsed at all—not even once. There is truth that, "we must give back to others what has been freely given to us," in order to keep the gifts of sobriety. To be of service is highly rewarding and fulfilling, based on my personal experience. It's a beautiful feeling to be able to see a fellow addict recover, grow, and flourish—especially when we have the power to help facilitate such a transformation.

"Service" is one aspect of the symbolic triangle found in 12-Step programs, indicating its value and importance toward long-term sobriety. Without service, the three-legged stool of Service, Unity, and Recovery, would inevitably crash and fall apart. It's crucial to my program to start serving the MA community. An important act of service includes attending and/or sharing in meetings.

Final thought: Today, I choose to be of service by sharing my experience, strength, and hope with my fellows.

February 22

Restored to Sanity

"Our insanity was evident as we repeated the same behavior over and over, yet somehow expected different results."

- *Life with Hope,* third edition, page 7

When I first entered the rooms of Marijuana Anonymous, what I wanted to know was how I could control my using, keeping it to parties or simply on weekends. The truth was, I wanted to know how to be happy and free which I had associated with getting high. The irony was that marijuana had not brought me any happiness or freedom, but rather pain and suffering at the end of my addiction.

The rooms of MA showed me a way out of this insanity and a new way of life. The program made me realize that marijuana was a means to an end, it was a desire to be free from the pain I felt inside. Working the 12 Steps, making a personal inventory, letting go of my character defects, and making amends for my past mistakes provided me the time to face this pain and move towards a life where I can be happy and free.

Final thought: Today, I remember the insanity of my addiction. I remember the pain of running away and remember to take a personal inventory, and when I am wrong, promptly admit it.

February 23

Fear vs. Faith

"We began to see the possibility that our beliefs...had been mistaken."

- Life with Hope, first edition, page 6

When I was younger, I lived in fear. I was afraid of so many things: anger, rejection, being unworthy, not being loved, not being good enough. I learned to speak very softly so that no one would notice me; then no one could be angry with me or reject me.

In early recovery I was talking with another MA member about fears. He told me that the opposite of fear is faith. My Higher Power is a god of love. I believed in my Higher Power but I thought that I had been forgotten about. I learned to trust my Higher Power and to know that I was always being cared for.

These days, I know that my Higher Power is watching over me and I can "let go and let God." I have faith in my Higher Power now. I am not afraid anymore because I know that my Higher Power is always there for me. I am so grateful for the gifts of my recovery and every day is a blessing.

Final thought: I will "let go and let God" today and every day.

February 24

Pause

"Gradually, as we listened to other recovering addicts, we became willing to do what was needed. We came to believe that a power greater than ourselves could restore us to sanity."

- Life with Hope, second edition, page 8-9

The most important thing I have been learning in recovery is, "this too shall pass." Every time an urge comes up to sabotage my recovery, or I feel desperate to make "the pain stop," I know that, gratefully, I have been given a moment to decide what to do; a pause, a moment of sanity, a moment of choice. I can work my program. I can call a fellow and they remind me in one way or another, "this too shall pass." My experience has shown me "it" always passes, whatever "it" is. It may not pass on my timeline but it always shifts as long as I am willing to work the tools of recovery and remember that it is OK to be temporarily uncomfortable.

This pause teaches me to pray, ask HP for help, call a fellow, feel the feeling, pause, wait, get into service, take a walk, trust the process and, most importantly, do not believe everything I think! The only way I am guaranteed to know "this too shall pass" is to remember I am not alone and to get out of my head and into my program. My recovery gives me this pause, this moment of choice, this restoration of sanity to choose. This too, no matter what, shall pass.

Final thought: Today, no matter what comes my way, I will remember, "this too shall pass." If I forget this, I will work my program, reach out to others and be grateful for the gift of this most important pause, this restoration to sanity that has been given to me.

February 25

Higher Power Showing Up

"For each step we take toward God, God takes a thousand steps toward us."

- Life with Hope, third edition, page 51

When I first came to Marijuana Anonymous, I understood God to be an all-knowing, judgmental, scary guy in the sky. I didn't like him very much, and I didn't think he cared for me either. I saw "God" in most of the Twelve Steps and thought, "I'll just skip that part." In meetings and conversations with my sponsor, I heard people talk about their Higher Power. For every person in the room, there was a different version of God. I read our literature that refers to a "loving," and "positive" Higher Power.

As I worked the Steps, I kept an "open mind and hopeful heart" (*Life with Hope* third edition, page 8). I took some time to think what I should call my Higher Power, since I wasn't too fond of the word God. Before I even had a name for it, my Higher Power started working in my life; I started to see how it was working in my life. It has always been there, I was just too stoned to notice. I started keeping track of "coincidences," and now I have a list of 50 ways my Higher Power has shown up in my life.

I don't believe in coincidences anymore. I believe that I'm in sync and cooperating with a divine, loving, kind, gentle, forgiving, humorous, beautiful universe, higher self, spirit family, master gardener, or cosmic parent. I am in awe every day and each day, and I thank MA for the gift of God, as I understand God.

Final thought: Today, I will take a step towards my Higher Power, by showing up at meetings, talking to other addicts, and practicing the spiritual principles of the Twelve Steps.

February 26

Figuring It Out

"The more we grow in this program, the more we realize that we know very little."

- *Life with Hope,* first edition, page 52

When I first got clean I thought I was too smart for this program. I found the slogans to be childish and simplistic. Sure, they say "one day at a time," but I know that really means I can never smoke again. I had it all "figured out" but in actuality I was too smart for my own good. I questioned all suggestions, thinking they didn't apply to me. My questions were not helping me to get this program.

I gradually learned to trust the process and the program. I no longer think of my "brilliant" mind as an asset. The longer I am sober the less I want to think and the more I want to feel. I have learned that the best thing I can do for my sobriety is to listen to my heart, rather than my monkey mind. "Figuring it out" is just another way to say "obsessing."

Final thought: Today, I will use my heart more than my head.

February 27

Willing to Believe

"There is room in MA for all beliefs or none. It doesn't matter if we are agnostic, atheist or theist. We all have a place here. There is no conflict. For each of us, a power greater than ourselves is whatever we choose it to be. It can be any positive, powerful thing that we are comfortable with."

- Life with Hope, first edition, page 9

When I first entered the rooms of MA and heard the word "God," I felt uncomfortable or hesitant to continue in the program. The word "God" carried a negative feeling due to my past messages from organized religion. However, when I listened to my fellows, I found that I could create my own Higher Power based on a new understanding of spirituality. I was told that I could come to believe in a loving, forgiving and compassionate Higher Power that would help remove the obsession to use marijuana as well as help me handle the complexities of recovery and my life. All I had to do was be willing to believe.

Final thought: Today, I will open my mind to a belief in a Power greater than myself. I am willing to believe that my Higher Power will restore me to sanity.

February 28

Letting Go of Perfectionism

"We began to see the possibility that our beliefs about ourselves, formed while using, had been mistaken."

- Life with Hope, second edition, page 6

I grew up in a pretty dysfunctional home, full of judgments and criticism. I thought I needed to be perfect to be loved, and that perfection was an attainable goal. It was a big relief to learn that there's no such thing as perfection. The readings tell me life is about "progress, not perfection." Another belief I grew up with was that I was alone, because I always felt alone. The first really big change in my recovery came the day I felt a presence and knew I wasn't alone. I figured it was my Higher Power and I spent four years trying to figure out what it was.

Finally, I came to the conclusion that it didn't matter what my Higher Power is—I just needed to believe there was a Higher Power that cared for me. I also heard from someone with decades of recovery that Higher Power is big, bigger than our human brains can comprehend. I'm free to believe whatever I want my Higher Power to look like, or just be an energy like love.

In recovery, I've learned that I'm not alone, and that actually I'm perfect just the way I am. After some years in recovery, I finally put down the hammer that I used to use to beat myself up with. As I let my Higher Power care for me, I care for myself."

Final thought: Today, I can accept that I'm a perfectly fine imperfect human being who is never alone.

February 29

Freedom from Addiction

"We were caught by the disease of addiction, ensnared in the insidious grip of marijuana."

- Life with Hope, first edition, page 2

Since I got clean, I've cultivated a healthy fear of marijuana. For years I was a slave to marijuana. I couldn't stop using, even though I wasn't getting high. I don't want pot to have one more day of my life. If I don't stay clean, I know I will lose all the gifts I have gained. Therefore, freedom from active addiction has to be the cornerstone of my life. I have a life today full of family, friends, love, work that I enjoy, and a sense of purpose. I can be of service today because I am clean and sober.

Final thought: Recovery has to be the top priority in my life today, if I want a life worth living.

March 1

As I Understood God

"We made a decision to have faith and began putting our trust in a power greater than ourselves."

- Life with Hope, first edition, page 12

When I first came into MA and realized there was the "God" word in the Steps, I really thought about getting up and walking out. It didn't take long before I realized that a lot of other folks in the meetings had a problem with that too. It wasn't that God; it was as I understand God. It could be my own understanding! The words "Higher Power" were meaningful to me. I appreciated that concept. I also liked that the gender was taken out of God. It was not God—He; maybe it was God—She; maybe it was God—It. It was as I understood God. It was a power greater than myself. For the first few years, the meetings and MA members were my Higher Power. We could do something together that I could not do alone. I'd tried too long.

As the years have gone by, my concept of God, Creator, Higher Power has had many definitions and/or concepts, and a great realization has come to me: I don't have to understand God! How could I? I am a small human on a small planet, in a small solar system, in an ordinary galaxy in a huge universe. When I see pictures of our galaxy, or nebulas, or other galaxies, I say, "There. That's God." Some small part of that huge God is what I think of as a loving, caring, parental God, who wants me to be a loving, caring person. That part of God, my part of God, wants me to be happy, loving, and serene; and that's the God I pray to. What are my prayers? There are really only two: "Help me, Help me, Help me," and "Thank you, Thank you, Thank you."

Final thought: Trusting my Higher Power cleared the way for my growth and recovery.

March 2

This Burden

"I have tried to control the uncontrollable for far too long. I ask that you take this burden from me."

- *Life with Hope,* first edition, page 13

Trying to push against doors that said "pull," wishing red lights were green, and wanting to be someone else in a different time and place were all symptoms of my "dis-ease." I thought if I prayed hard enough, things would change. When that didn't work, I would pout and become angry. The peace-loving beatnik disappeared. Recovery has taught me there's an easier, gentler way.

Final thought: God can relieve the self-imposed burden of needing control. All I need is acceptance and willingness.

March 3

"You Know, Guilt Sucks!"

"...the most important aspects of the Fifth Step are the acceptance, compassion, and forgiveness we feel from our sponsor and from a Higher Power. The guilty feelings born in our past start to fall away."

- Life with Hope, first edition, page 23

I was in shock the first time my sponsor uttered that phrase to me. I spent half my Fourth Step ruminating over tragedies: my errors in judgment, the colossal mistakes I'm still paying for, and regrets I've carried with me forever. It never failed when any of my indiscretions surfaced, the "poor me" pose would emerge, the antacids would pop out and my favorite flight response would take over—"run, baby run."

My sponsor would always tell me, with his kind truth—able to cut to the chase, "Why let your ego run havoc through your life? It's all a mind game anyway, a big cosmic joke. The ego wants to keep you in its clutches until it's time to take your dirt nap then it'll keep on haunting you way into your next life. Trick the ego and don't buy into the guilt—take responsibility, 'fess up to your wrongs, make those sincere amends, then move on with your life. Don't worry, don't compound the mess, there will be more mistakes that will follow. For God's sake, we're only human."

Final thought: Guilt rides the coattails of the ego. It's time for a new wardrobe.

March 4

Gentle Guidance

"By staying in the present, we release the past and let go of the future... to release our self-will, we make a decision to turn our will and our lives over to the care of a higher power."

- *MA Workbook*, first edition, 11th printing, page 9

To help me stay in the present, I have my own version of the Step Three prayer. One of my favorite prompts in our workbook is the invitation to craft our own version of the prayer. Mine goes like this:

> I'm grateful for another day
>
> For peace in my own heart I pray.
>
> May inspiration be the light
>
> That guides my morning, day and night.
>
> May life unfold in its own time
>
> And gently show the path that's mine.

Where I once willfully swung my machete wildly through the gnarly vines of a dark jungle, I can now envision a beautiful meadow, where the soft grass and beds of clover part before my feet to show me the way. Turning my will and life over to the care of my Higher Power means accepting an invitation to live a life of creativity and wonder. I am so, so glad that I made this decision!

Final thought: Today, I choose to be guided not by impulse or instinct, but by intuition and inspiration.

March 5

Evolving Idea of Higher Power

"We were taught that a little willingness goes a long way towards building faith."

- Life with Hope, second edition, page 12

Early in recovery, I recoiled at any mention of God or a Higher Power. It didn't make sense to me. After a short while, I realized that people who had what I wanted, had some kind of Higher Power. At first, I acted as if I had a Higher Power. The first time I did a Third Step, I imagined my Higher Power as two oak trees, and I laid in a hammock held by these two trees. I suppose trees were my first Higher Power. Various different imaginings later, my idea of Higher Power is more of an energetic force that moves life in our universe. I want to surrender to the glorious mystery that holds us up on this spinning planet. When I think of Higher Power that way, I am comforted and feel secure.

Faith takes practice. I read recently that faith, like everything else, comes and goes, which was reassuring. On the days I don't feel a connection, I know that it is an illusion, because I am always connected to everything. Lately, talking out loud to the air around me, I choose to believe that something is hearing me. I am reminded that there's something bigger than me that supports me. I heard early on in my recovery that "the power within me is far greater than any fear before me," which is another comforting message.

Final thought: Today, I will include my Higher Power in more of my actions and decisions today. I am willing to receive divine guidance.

March 6

Spiritual Journey

"Recovery...is a process, not an event."

- Life with Hope, first edition, page 4

When I first started attending Marijuana Anonymous meetings, I thought that I would get "recovered" in about six months and then I would be able to smoke marijuana like a "regular" person. I actually thought that I would celebrate my six months clean time by smoking a joint! A friend told me that this was not the way to celebrate my recovery. I listened to my friend and I celebrated by continuing to go to MA meetings instead.

I discovered that those in Marijuana Anonymous would love me until I loved myself. Now my best friends are my recovery friends and they have enhanced my life. I diligently worked the Steps with my sponsor. This helped me establish a strong foundation for my recovery. Slowly, I was able to let go of the guilt and shame of the past, which had limited my spiritual growth. I now realize that while I was using, I wasn't growing. I was just hanging on to the old thoughts and fears.

My recovery journey was difficult sometimes, but every event was an opportunity for growth. This required work, but now I have a greater spiritual connection. Recovery saved my life and I am so grateful to my Higher Power. Now, I am able to be my true self. My life is happy now; I feel at peace. I am so grateful that I have trudged this "road of happy destiny."

Final thought: Today and every day, I thank my Higher Power for another day clean and sober. I am so grateful!

March 7

Perseverance

"We had spent our entire lives and our using careers based on self-centeredness. This attitude does not change overnight. It is a lifelong process requiring the practice of perseverance."

- Life with Hope, first edition, page 33

In active addiction, I was willing to do whatever it took to ensure my marijuana supply would never run out. In the past, at times, weed was hard to obtain but I always made sure I had some stashed away at all times. I would even lie to friends about it so I could smoke their stash instead.

Now, I try to apply that same level of determination to my recovery. I will give my sobriety as much time and energy as I gave my addiction. I will make myself go to a meeting, especially when I do not want to. If there is no in-person MA meeting, I will seek online or phone meetings. Twelve Step meetings are never hard to find. Other fellowships also have a lot to offer.

I smoked pot every day, so why shouldn't I attend a meeting every day? Attending meetings and helping other addicts is akin to getting vaccinated against relapse. The immunity will last for up to 24 hours, and then I require another booster. In order to experience a daily reprieve, I must be willing to go to any length to help fellow addicts.

I will persevere even when it hurts. I was told that pain is the touchstone of spiritual growth because pain is just weakness leaving the body. One day at a time, I am willing to do whatever it takes to maintain my sobriety as guided by my Higher Power.

Final thought: Today, I will embrace the pain; as an expression of my gratitude for the gifts I do have, I will persevere.

March 8

Belief and Faith

"This minimum of belief is enough to open the door and cross the threshold. Once we are on the other side, our belief and trust in a Higher Power broadens and deepens as we continue taking the Steps."

- Life with Hope, third edition, page 9

In Step Two, it says "came to believe," not "now I believe", or, "I wouldn't need any more Steps." "Came" is a verb; a verb is an action, a movement; so it's a movement towards something, in this case, towards belief, towards sanity, and spirituality. I get to know God, just like getting to know a new friend; it happens over time. I don't instantly know everything about someone the first time I meet them. I build that relationship and take actions to get closer to them.

I make a decision in Step Three to clear the lines and the path to get to know my HP, to give my HP a chance to introduce itself to me. To make a decision to turn over my will and my life in Step Three—without quite knowing exactly what my Higher Power is—I took a leap of faith. "Even if we do not understand or feel connected to a Higher Power, it is possible to work Step Three." (*MA Workbook,* first edition, 11th printing, page 9)

Final thought: To take Steps Two and Three, I do not have to understand and define my Higher Power. I only have to be open to the process of relinquishing self-will and taking the actions of the Steps to deepen my connection and understanding of my Higher Power.

March 9

Courage to Face the Truth

"We had tried everything over the years to change reality, to no avail. In MA we at last found the courage to face the truth."

- *Life with Hope,* first edition, page 3

Sobriety requires courage. The Fourth through Eleventh Steps require me to examine myself and my patterns and relationships. They require me to hold myself accountable for being the version of myself that I can be proud of, and to let go of the things I have burdened myself with that were not mine to bear. There are two types of pain: the type that comes from growth, and the type that comes from betraying myself. One of these two types of pain is optional.

Being clean gives me a clear head to choose for myself, through my spiritual work, which pain I allow to continue in my life. I am gentle and kind with myself as I go through the growing pains of becoming my truest version of myself. I release myself from the denial of what I know to be true, and take action to create a more authentic life for myself. This is the most beautiful gift of sobriety: connecting with myself, and in turn, allowing others to connect with me.

Final thought: Today, I will choose to honor the truth within myself and will do so with a clear mind as a result of my sobriety.

March 10

The Power of Faith

"The power of faith gives our lives a new direction."

- Life with Hope, first edition, page 13

When I first heard the word "faith" in MA, I was completely broken and believed in nothing, especially not myself. The religious connotations behind the words were all that I noticed and, due to my fractured relationship with organized religion, I recoiled at the very mention of it. Today, I have a much better understanding of what faith means in my life. Having started at a place of self-loathing, paranoia, isolation, and cynicism; I got to sobriety, serenity, and security.

This transformation came about through faith that not only could things get better for me, but most importantly that I deserved them to get better. Today, I have faith in my Higher Power's guidance and will for me, as well as faith in others. My insecurity has been replaced with self-esteem.

Final thought: Faith rebuilt me from the inside out and gave me back my self-esteem. Today, I am happy just to be me.

March 11

Responsible Decisions

"We found that by deciding to turn our will and lives over to the care of God, *as we each understood God*, our lives and the responsible use of our freedom to choose were returned to us."

- Life with Hope, third edition, page 12

When I was actively using, there was no room for a Higher Power in my life, let alone faith in one. My self-will controlled me and led me to make many poor decisions. These decisions depleted my self-esteem, harmed my relationships, cost me financially, and ultimately sent me into deep depression, suicidal thoughts, and stays in the hospital.

When I accepted my powerlessness, became willing to believe in a Higher Power that could restore me to sanity, and made a decision to turn my will and my life over to the care of God, as I understood God, I finally realized that I could give up my fruitless attempts to control things. I could leave in God's hands the things over which I have no control. "Turning it over" allows me to focus on the few things I can control, and faith in my Higher Power gives me the freedom to make wise and responsible choices in my life.

Final thought: God, today help me to remember that your loving care and guidance are always with me, and that by turning over my will and my life to you, I am free to make the wise decisions that help me to live my best life.

March 12

Faith Guides Me

"As we loosen our grip on the reins of our lives, we find we are being led, slowly and certainly, in the right direction—towards home."

- *Life with Hope,* second edition, page 57

I was forced to let go of the reins of my life. This program did not allow me to keep holding on the way I was while I lived in active addiction. In order to take the Twelve Steps, I had to let go absolutely to find home and serenity within myself. Once I learned to let go, I found I was being guided by my Higher Power and each time that I let go, I was guided further.

I lost my job during the pandemic of 2020 and after two days of crying and screaming at myself, I finally picked up the 800-pound phone. The fellow I called told me the job that I was now searching for was also searching for me. It was a true God shot. I had not thought of looking for work in this way. I looked at employment like it was a prize to be won. The fellow made me realize my place of employment will be just as lucky to have me as I am to have them.

God is leading me in the right direction when I pray. Every night I pray for God to guide me; to guide my actions, my voice, my thoughts and feelings. I meditate on the here and now. It is the most blissful part of my day. Sometimes I receive answers from my Higher Power during my meditation that I am truly blessed to know. Finding a job isn't easy. I will take many Steps in order to find the right fit. I have faith that God is on my side and is looking out for me with every Step I take.

Final thought: Today, meditation and prayer are an everyday regimen that saves me from catastrophizing and brings me peace.

March 13

Our Community

"...the group is more powerful than any of its individual members..."

- *Life with Hope,* first edition, page 7

God knows us in our loneliness. We know God better in our togetherness. Some say sobriety isn't recovery, and that recovery is being in community. Fellow recovering addicts restore my faith so that I can stay sober. They help me, sometimes because I ask, and sometimes without my knowing it. To experience these things though, I must be with others. When using, I isolated. All I could see was myself and that was the last thing I wanted to look at. Today, when I'm with others, I have the chance to be of service and I give them the opportunity to be of service. When I listen, I swear I can hear God speaking, and when I'm hugged, I can feel God's arms. When I share honestly and act with integrity, my shame and guilt continue to melt away. I don't need to hide and I can see so much more than just myself.

Final thought: With sobriety, I have the ability to act like a polished lens, fully transparent, to magnify God's love so that others may see it more clearly.

March 14

Faith—The Opposite of Fear

"We began to transform our fears into faith and started to find a new way to love—unconditionally."

- Life with Hope, first edition, page 20

I had many fears when I was younger. I was afraid of anger; I was afraid of rejection; I was afraid of abandonment; I was afraid that people didn't like me; I was afraid to speak up. These fears led to a lack of self-esteem, a feeling of being unworthy. I learned to live in my own fantasy world where I wouldn't have to face these fears. Smoking marijuana seemed to enhance my fantasy world and I could forget about all of my problems. However, I soon realized that getting high was a way to avoid facing my problems. I thought that I was helping my depression by getting high but, actually, my depression increased to the point that I became suicidal. I was hospitalized and had to face reality.

When I entered the rooms of Marijuana Anonymous, I found that I was loved and accepted just the way I was. I remember hearing that fear is the opposite of faith. I learned if I had faith in my Higher Power, if I asked to do my Higher Power's will, that my Higher Power would always be there for me. Before I entered recovery and had become so unhappy, I thought that my Higher Power had forgotten about me. Now, I know that I had been mistaken and that I had always been under God's care. Now, I believe the direction that my life takes is always what is best for me, even if I don't realize it at the time.

Final thought: Today and always, I am grateful for the blessings in my life and for my recovery.

March 15

Turning It Over

"By starting to trust our Higher Power, we cleared the way for growth and recovery. Now we no longer have to rely on the weak force of self-will to solve our problems. Faith and acceptance are our new solutions. The power of faith gives our lives a new direction."

- Life with Hope, third edition, page 13

I was raised to believe people could do anything they set their minds to. Self-will, seen as the most powerful force in the world, was the cornerstone of this belief. While I had many successes in life as a result of pushing against the odds, I met my match with cannabis. No matter how hard I tried to control my use, I found my will was powerless in the struggle. Only when I accepted the fact that I was an addict and reached out in faith for help did things begin to change.

As I began to recognize other areas in my life where I was powerless, which I had to turn over to my Higher Power, I gradually began to experience an empowering new faith and the clarity that comes with it. In the years of struggling with the parts of my life over which I had no control, I had neglected, in that struggle, the crucial aspects of my life over which I did have power.

By letting go of that over which I have no control, I have more time, energy, and power to be responsible to work on those things I can control. In this process, my faith is strengthened, my clarity is sharpened, and those things I once thought impossible now materialize, often effortlessly, as I find God is doing for me what I could never do for myself.

Final thought: Today, I will practice faith in my life, doing my best work and leaving the results to my Higher Power.

March 16

Facing My Fears

"Higher Power...Grant me honesty, courage, humility, and serenity, to face that which keeps me from you and others."

- Life with Hope, first edition, page 13

I don't ask my Higher Power to keep me clean, or to make my life better, or to make my problems go away. I ask for honesty, courage, humility, and serenity. Fear kept me from my Higher Power. I was afraid to give myself to God, afraid to be vulnerable with others, afraid to let go of control, afraid to love or be loved, afraid to fail and afraid to succeed!

As I kept working through the Steps, I kept facing those fears, with the support of my sponsor and the other people in MA. As I continue to face those fears, they keep getting smaller because Step Four helped me to recognize them for what they are: fleeting thoughts and feelings that don't define me. Step Six helped me understand how they keep me from my Higher Power and others and aren't effective in leading a clean and spiritual life. Step Seven helps me pray to have them removed, which I think of as seeing through them. Step Eleven helps me stay close to my God so those fears just keep getting smaller and smaller. Step Twelve gets me out of myself completely; out of fear and into love and service for others. I am blessed with actual times in my life when I live in love rather than fear.

Final thought: Today, I will ask for help in facing my fears so that I may learn from them, see through, and overcome them. I will ask to be closer to my Higher Power, others, and love.

March 17

Choices on Recovery's Trail

"Step Three asked us to make a decision based upon our acceptance of our addiction and powerlessness that we had identified in Steps One and Two. Before, we alternated between being controlling or controlled."

- Life with Hope, third edition, page 11

Embers fade with glowing light.

Addictions die with mighty fight.

Our souls rekindled with a renewed pact.

With backs upright and shoulders back,

We walk among the clear of mind.

Dreams return our thoughts in kind.

Our purpose walks a straightened rail.

New life awaits on recovery's trail.

Final thought: Today, my choices in life are guided by my Higher Power. I no longer walk alone.

March 18

Belief in a Higher Power

"It is not necessary to acquire a major God consciousness to be able to cease using. All we need is to maintain an open mind and a hopeful heart. It is not necessary to say yes. It is, however, important to stop saying *no*."

- Life with Hope, first edition, page 7

In my compulsive use of pot I had become incredibly isolated from the world; I kept saying "no" to opportunities presented by life. I recognized that I was powerless over marijuana and began my recovery. The final sentence in this passage became my personal slogan and guiding principle under which my life opened up to the world again.

Final thought: Today, I practice the principles of open-mindedness and hope.

March 19

Making a Decision

"The humility of asking for help keeps us from self-righteousness and protects us against outbreaks of either grandiosity or self-pity."

- Life with Hope, first edition, page 51

In Step Three, we made a decision to turn our will and our lives over to the care of a Higher Power of our understanding. At this Step, I struggled to understand what it meant to turn my will and my life over to the care of a Higher Power. I was still stuck in patterns of thinking in extremes; it had to be all or nothing, right?

Luckily, my sponsor pointed out that all I was asked to do was to make a decision. I was asked to have faith that a power greater than myself could possibly guide and direct me. I was asked to be empowered to trust in a higher force of energy, purpose, and love that is always streaming through me and around me. I was not asked to submit. I was asked to take action with the gifts my Higher Power had imparted upon me.

I was not expected to be a perfect human being, just one who is willing to connect to new solutions in life. A relationship with a Higher Power is infinitely available to me. I sit in meditation; walk in the woods; and reach out and tune in to the frequency of the source of my Higher Power.

Final thought: Today, I get to actively decide to channel my energy, to learn and grow in a daily relationship to a spiritual connection that speaks the language of my heart and spirit.

March 20

There Is No Definition

"Higher Power, I have tried to control the uncontrollable for far too long. I ask that you take this burden from me. I acknowledge that my life is unmanageable. I ask for your care and guidance."

- *Life with Hope,* second edition, page 13

My relationship with a Higher Power is a fundamental part of my recovery. I'm freed from the need for control and I gain strength knowing that my Higher Power loves me unconditionally. It is a powerful positive energy that I truly believe wants to help me, teach me, and lead me towards becoming my best self. I do not understand what my Higher Power is, or how it does things. All I have to do is show up, follow through on my responsibilities, and be kind to myself and others. I get to trust that Higher Power will take care of the rest.

My life when I was using marijuana was disorganized, hollow, and repetitive. My addiction kept me from being social and being present in my life. I feel blessed to be in recovery and to be fully present each and every day.

I came to the program, like many others, without a belief in a Higher Power. I was never against it, but I never knew that it could be anything of my own understanding. I can choose to believe in whatever works best for me because it allows me to let go, and go with the flow. I can fully enjoy each and every moment without obsessively holding on or pushing things away.

MA is a community; a power greater than myself. My friendships here have taught me so much about healthier ways to live and relate. It has truly transformed my life into something that I look forward to every night when I go to sleep.

Final thought: Today, I am excited to be myself. I've become patient enough to recognize that everything is on God's time, not my own.

March 21

How Can I Be of Service?

"There is no satisfaction greater than knowing that one has made an honest attempt to help another, regardless of the results."

- Life with Hope, first edition, page 64

Sometimes I think, "Why me? Why does this have to happen to me?" But, I know that the experiences I go through only teach me to become a stronger, better person. These trials and tribulations are necessary to grow in order to get through any situation and be of service. Is there strength in your faith to get through the situation? Ask each day what you can do for another. "How can I be of service? Please show me what I can do for the addict that is still sick," I ask this each morning in my meditations. Being of service is one part of the MA triangle. There were times when I took on too much. I take my commitments very seriously.

Here is a story I like: A sponsee and a sponsor were having breakfast. The sponsee asked, "What is the difference between being of service and having a commitment?" The Sponsor looked down at the plate and said, "You see these ham and eggs? The chicken was of service, the pig made a commitment."

Final thought: Today, I ask how can I be of service and help another addict.

March 22

Letting Go

"It was the beginning of learning how to 'turn it over' and to 'let go and let God'..."

- *Life with Hope,* second edition, page 13

We've all been amazed by the skill of the gymnast who flips over from one bar to another or marveled at the trapeze artist swinging freely in midair. I've come to believe in a similar leap of faith. For many years I held on hopelessly to my addiction to marijuana. I endlessly swung between the false high and the desperate lows. Admitting that I was powerless over pot required a belief in something other than myself; something bigger. I couldn't do it alone. I had to let go of the bar of addiction and trust that there would be another to hang on to.

In recovery, I've come up against many moments which require this trust: changing relationships, job loss, the death of loved ones. Rather than hanging on to that pain and trying to smoke it away, I've learned to let go and let God.

Final thought: Let the bar come to you and learn to participate with grace in flying free from addiction.

March 23

The Mask

"We humbly accepted who we had been, and who we were becoming."

- Life with Hope, first edition, page 45

When I was using, I hid behind a mask. Smoking marijuana was a secret that I kept from others. On the outside, I thought that I looked like a "normal" person, but inside I hid my demons. I had a lot of fear and this fear helped to create my mask and keep it in place. I thought that I could protect my inner self. I thought that this mask would prevent others from seeing my suffering. I was smiling even though I was suffering from depression, because I didn't want anyone to know how unhappy I was. I thought that smoking marijuana would let me forget about my troubles. I thought that I felt better when I was high.

In recovery, I found out that these thoughts and feelings were a delusion. Smoking marijuana had only intensified my depression. By trying to escape my negative feelings, they only worsened. I was afraid of rejection but I found the courage to let go of my mask. With my recovery, I am able to accept myself just the way I am. I have learned that I am lovable; my Higher Power loves me. I have learned that I don't have to hide my feelings; I can be seen as my true self.

Final thought: I don't need a mask anymore; I can let the real me shine through.

March 24

Happy, Joyous, and Free

"As a result of this step, we begin to experience contentment, serenity, and fulfillment."

- Life with Hope, second edition, page 60

Ever since I entered recovery, I've heard it said that our Higher Power wants us to be happy, joyous, and free. While I've repeated that phrase often, I haven't always lived it. A friend who knew a lot about the brain explained to me that we have grooves in our brain where old ideas reside, and by using affirmations, I can raise the grooves, and not fall into old beliefs. One of my old beliefs is that if other people are suffering, then it's not OK for me to be happy. I know intellectually that my suffering does not decrease another's suffering, but that doesn't always help me to not suffer.

Just like I make a decision every day to turn my will and my life over to my Higher Power, I have found that I need to make a similar decision to be happy, joyous, and free. My old ideas need reminders that it's good for my well-being to be happy, joyous, and free. When I feel joyous, I am kinder to other people, and kinder to myself.

Final thought: Today, I know it's good for me to be happy, joyous, and free.

March 25

Turning Over Self-Will

"Step Three called us into action, for it was only by action that self-will could be removed."

- *Life with Hope,* first edition, page 11

This is a program of action, and the action suggested by this Step is enormous. I find that in order to make change manageable, I have to break it down into tangible actions. Each day is filled with moments when I may fall into my self-will, and each of those moments is an opportunity to instead do my Higher Power's will.

Final thought: Today, in those moments, I find that I can turn my will over by repeating the Third Step Prayer, having a moment of quiet reflection, or simply asking, "What is the right thing to do?"

March 26

Living in the Present

"If we have been diligent, honest and painstaking in our recovery, the tools we have acquired in this program will come to our aid when we meet life's serious challenges..."

- Life with Hope, first edition, page 67

Living just for today relieves the burden of the past and the fear of the future. I learned to take whatever actions are necessary and to leave the results in the hands of my Higher Power. In my active addiction, fear of the future and what might happen was a reality for me. "What if I got arrested?" "Lost my jobs?" "My spouse died?" "What if I went bankrupt?" It was not unusual for me to spend hours, even days thinking about what might happen. I played out entire conversations and scenarios before they ever occurred, then charted my course on the basis of "what if." By doing this, I set myself up for disappointment after disappointment.

From listening in meetings, I learn to live in the present, not the prophecies of doom and gloom. I can only deal with what is real today, not my fearful fantasies of the future. Coming to believe that my Higher Power has only the best in store for me is one way I can combat that fear. I hear at meetings that my Higher Power won't give me more than what I can handle in one day. I know from experience that if I ask, the God I've come to understand will surely care for me. I stay clean and sober through adverse situations by practicing my faith in the care of a Power greater than myself. Each time I do, I become less fearful of "what if" and more comfortable with what is.

Final thought: Today, I will look forward to the future with faith in my Higher Power.

March 27

The Freedom to Choose

"We found that by deciding to turn our will and lives over to the care of God, as we each understood God, our lives and the responsible use of our freedom to choose were returned to us."

- Life with Hope, second edition, page 13

The freedom to choose; what a foreign concept that was! I had convinced myself that I was choosing to use marijuana, but marijuana was using me. Marijuana had me in her grips and wrapped me in chains that I could not escape. It wasn't until I did Step Three with my sponsor and made the decision to turn my will and life over to the care of God, that I discovered newfound freedom; freedom that was rejuvenating, refreshing, and lifesaving. It broke the chains. The merry-go-round from hell that was my insidious marijuana addiction stopped spinning.

I was able to make the decision to get off that ride thus ending my suffering. Slowly but surely, my life got better. The fog lifted; the healing began. It doesn't stop there though; I have to make the daily decision to turn my will over to God. Every morning, I set aside time to pray and meditate, that's when I talk to God and remind myself that I am not in control, that thy will be done. If I don't do that, I will quickly try to control every aspect of my day and when doing so, I create chaos, disappointment, stress, and worry. It also pours over into wanting to control other people; talk about disappointment and frustration!

I am still human so I don't do this perfectly, but every moment that I am clean I get to try. Step Three alleviates the pain and sorrow I so often inflicted on myself. The good news is that I don't have to live that way anymore. I am recovering, one Step, one decision, one choice, one day at a time.

Final thought: Today, I have the freedom to choose, and I choose to turn my will and life over to the care of God.

March 28

Progress Not Perfection

"When we strive for perfection, our ego gets in the way of letting our Higher Power into our recovery."

- MA Workbook, first edition, page 41

One of my character defects is perfectionism. I used to think that was a good thing. Why wouldn't I want everything I do to be perfect? When I came into MA, though, I learned that my perfectionism was an ego trip rooted in fear. My fear of not being perfect meant I avoided activities and ventures if I thought I couldn't be the absolute best. Instead of gauging my interests and joys by my own deepest values, I compared myself to others and gave undue credence to what others (or, more likely, what I thought others) thought of me. This led me to avoid life's challenges, resist engaging in new activities, or to take risks in my career, because if I couldn't do it perfectly, why bother? When I did engage in something new or challenging, I was plagued by fear of failure. I would often freeze or procrastinate in anticipation of results I was convinced would be subpar and inadequate.

Of course, getting high was a great way to check out and avoid the feelings of self-loathing and disappointment this approach to life produced. Now, thanks to working MA's program, I look forward to trying new things and taking reasonable risks, because I know that I only have to do what's right in front of me, and my Higher Power will handle the outcomes. I trust that God has the perfect plan for me, and I don't have to be more than me, with all the ups and downs, character assets and defects, successes and setbacks that being human entails— one day at a time.

Final thought: Today, I strive for progress, not perfection.

March 29

Emotional Maturity/Gratitude

"Our new attitudes bring about self-esteem, inner strength and serenity that is not easily shaken by any of life's hard times."

- *Life with Hope,* first edition, page 68

I grew up as an insecure, shy, lonely child. I learned to disappear in the background; I had no self-esteem. I was fearful. Smoking marijuana alleviated these fears at first. I wasn't afraid to talk to others and I felt like I was accepted. I didn't realize that this was a temporary feeling; soon I became very paranoid and I withdrew. Depression became part of my daily life.

I was desperate when I came to MA; I was broken. I was surprised at how much I was welcomed into the rooms. I struggled at first. With the help of my sponsor, my Higher Power and my friends in MA, I was able to stop smoking marijuana and find a new way of living. As I worked the Steps and embraced my recovery, my depression lessened and I became stronger. I realized that I was an acceptable, lovable person. I could let go of my fear with the help of my Higher Power. The lessons of the Twelve Steps have become part of my life and the tools of recovery help me when I have challenges in my life. I can look at problems as "growth opportunities." I look to my Higher Power for guidance. I am able to be of service and help others. I found inner peace and serenity. I am "happy, joyous and free" and I am so grateful for my recovery which has changed my life.

Final thought: Today, I will live by faith, not fear, and reach out to others.

March 30

Getting "Right Sized"

"The basic ingredients of humility are unpretentiousness and a willingness to submit to a Higher Power's will."

- Life with Hope, second edition, page 31

When I got to recovery and heard the term "humility," I had no idea what they were talking about. I had to look the word up in the dictionary. It still didn't make sense until I started working the Steps with my sponsor. I kept hearing people at meetings say things like humility is being "right size" with your Higher Power (and other people), not better than or worse than. I also heard that the Latin root of the word humility means "of the earth." I heard that addicts are ego-maniacs with an inferiority complex.

As I worked the Steps, I began to lose that sense of feeling "less than" all the time. A miracle happened and I began to work the Third Step every day, praying to my Higher Power to do their will, not mine. Being in acceptance also feels like humility because it means I know I'm not in charge or thinking I know best.

Final thought: Today, I know I can be right sized, not better than or worse than.

March 31

Living by Faith

"Learning to live by faith took practice; it opened the way to a new reliance on a Higher Power and the restoration of our inner wisdom. The turning point for us was the decision to relinquish control."

- Life with Hope, third edition, page 13

When I started my recovery I was sure that I could do this by myself. I was a strong, smart, and intelligent person; this wouldn't be too hard; all I had was a problem with smoking marijuana. I didn't have much faith in these Steps or trust in a sponsor. Yet, I kept slipping and relapsing and my life was more unmanageable than ever before.

Finally, I had to admit that I didn't know much about recovery and I couldn't do this by myself. I had to finally get honest, and try turning my will over to a power greater than myself however I choose to visualize it. The more I practice this tool of recovery, the more I have faith that this is working better than my way of doing it.

I've heard it said that my will is what I "want" to do, and God's will is what I "need" to do. Time and time again things that used to baffle me became easier to manage. The choices I started to make were no longer based on self-will but on how I could be helpful to others. When I stopped trying to drive the bus, I started to enjoy the ride.

Final thought: Today, I place my faith in the program of recovery and in the hands of my Higher Power.

April 1

Letting Go of the Past

"We held on to resentments about the past which prohibited us from embracing the present and living our lives to the fullest. Some of us were full of remorse and could not forgive ourselves for making mistakes. That is, we would not accept our humanity."

- Life with Hope, first edition, page 16

Taking my Fourth Step inventory was a difficult process. I had people who had wronged me that I never wanted to forgive, and others who I wished I had never wronged. I had previously thought that the answer to resentment and remorse was to push them far into the recesses of my mind, and bottle up any negative emotions I experienced as a result of them. I realized that by trying to ignore them, I was actually giving them more power over me. I could not let those feelings continue to dominate my life. I had to forgive people who had wronged me, not for them but for myself. I had to forgive myself for my own wrongdoings. No amount of anger or regret is going to change the past, but I can change my attitude going forward. I can acknowledge that without my past, I wouldn't be where I am in the present.

Final thought: Today, I will be grateful for who I am right now, instead of regretting who I was in the past.

April 2

The Fellowship

"...practically everyone can easily and naturally draw strength and support from the fellowship."

- *Life with Hope,* first edition, page 7

Getting to know other recovering addicts can extend outside the rooms and the meetings. Often the newcomer can share more directly and inclusively in our deepening experience and explore new concepts like compassion, strength, and hope. This is one way of showing gratitude and it blesses not only us but those with whom we share it. Minds are opened to new possibilities of hope over despair. When I start understanding that we do together what we cannot do alone, I awaken my consciousness to a powerful spirit of unity. A trail has been blazed for us to follow and, together, we can proceed in a Good Orderly Direction (i.e. God.) Those gentle warriors that blazed this trail have led by example and, when we care and share our new way of life, we honor their spirits.

Faith allows me to be fully present with fellow addicts in whom I trust and who trust me. Honesty becomes second nature. I live fully, love wastefully, and become what my Higher Power means me to be. It becomes less about me and more about us as we grow our spirit and reach out to newcomers and to addicts who still suffer. I become music, soar to new heights, and become so encompassed in faith that I illuminate new trails I could never have imagined as I walked in the darkness. You might read all this and say, "Whoa, easy does it—I just wanna quit weed!" This is where recovery begins. Because I've been there, I can tell you that a whole new life awaits you; just start following some simple Steps.

Final thought: Today, you can trust your heart to something that can help you do the impossible. It is suggested that we just show up, be consciously present, and have faith by opening ourselves to a Higher Power.

April 3

"We Do, and Then We Understand"—Patience and Action

"We were taught that a little willingness goes a long way towards building faith. Most of us resisted. We tried to understand this Step before we made the decision to have faith and act upon it."

- Life with Hope, third edition, page 12

When I enter the rooms of recovery, I see the gifts of sobriety blossoming in my fellows' lives. I see their serenity, their joy, the even-keeled ways they respond to "life on life's terms." I want that for myself, and I begin working the program earnestly, attending meetings, reading literature, and working with a sponsor. I may feel frustrated or discouraged when the serenity and security I have witnessed in others doesn't immediately manifest in my life. I must remind myself that I am in it for the long haul.

The knowledge and experiences through which I attain physical, emotional, and spiritual recovery are forged through this process. I can't fast-forward to the end and expect results. As the saying goes, "We don't think our way to right action. We act our way to right thinking." I do, and then I understand.

There might be days when I feel jaded or disheartened but straying from this path risks leaving before the miracle happens. I put my faith in the program and in my Higher Power, turn to my sponsor and fellows, and try to act my way to right thinking until I experience the serenity and joy I first saw in others.

Final thought: Today, I prioritize acting in alignment with my recovery without seeking immediate results.

April 4

What a Relief!

"We were living the illusion of control, thinking we could control not only our using, but also other people, places, and things."

- *Life with Hope,* first edition, page 1

I began my recovery unwilling to continue using marijuana to "solve" all my problems, but also reluctant to work on myself or to confess my long-held secrets. I desired the serenity, self-confidence, and maturity which others in the rooms seemed to have, but I didn't want to do the work in order to obtain those things. I figured I could do it my way and be just as well off. "Be of service?" What? "Get a sponsor?" No way. "Work the Steps?" Unnecessary! Staying clean was enough for me, and I considered my abstinence to be real "recovery."

After six months of not using, my mind was still racing. I obsessed about everything under the sun. I felt like a fraud sitting in meetings without taking the most basic suggestions. It was time to surrender! I finally asked a member with more time in the fellowship to sponsor me.

Final thought: Today, I will remember that God has a plan for this world which doesn't involve me in the driver's seat. I can let go of the steering wheel and enjoy the ride. Whee!

April 5

Cross Addiction

"The entire foundation of our program depends upon an honest admission of our powerlessness over addiction..."

- Life with Hope, first edition, page 3

Stopping my use of marijuana freed me from the hell of my marijuana abuse, but it did not free me from the hell of addiction. While the initial reprieve from stopping marijuana was powerful enough to allow me to start working the Steps, making big changes in my life, chairing meetings, and even taking on a few sponsees, I hit another bottom and ended up in treatment for a behavior that had become completely beyond my control.

This helped me realize that addiction was not simply limited to drug use, but could manifest in powerful behavioral patterns. Moreover, it allowed me to finally recognize that the problem was not the drug or the behaviors, the problem was in me. While thankfully this program adheres to a singleness of purpose concept that allowed me to connect with other marijuana addicts and cease my marijuana use, my addiction had a much more powerful hold than I ever could have imagined.

It took me almost half a decade to realize that my marijuana use was a symptom of a much bigger problem—and without addressing the trauma, negative self-talk, resentments, judgment, and self-deceit/manipulation that were festering under the surface, my addiction had never really departed, but simply went into hibernation until it found another set of vices on which to manifest, arguably even stronger than before.

I ultimately had to realize that I had been lying to myself. Although I had stopped using marijuana and was an active member of a 12-Step program, was I fully in recovery? The painful truth is that I was an addict who had stopped using marijuana and then tried to justify and rationalize that this was enough for me to stay healthy.

Final thought: Today, I will be honest with myself. Is there something that I am doing in excess worth examining that may be feeding my addiction?

April 6

A Big Life

"The people in MA seemed to have a long-term solution to the problem of marijuana addiction. I wanted what they had."

- I Came to Life, Life with Hope, third edition, page 108

When I walked into these rooms I was sure that I was Not an addict. I thought I had a great Big Life. I thought I was a hard worker in an industry that I loved. I thought I had an amazing lifestyle. I thought that I was the life of the party and had so many friends. I thought I had it all and I thought that I lost it all when I hit rock bottom. Not once had it occurred to me that I lost it all because I was high from when I woke up to when I went to bed. I really wasn't doing my best work. I worked just hard enough to get by and stay high. I always left those friends or they left me when the weed was gone. I was alone and lonely and I didn't even know it.

I walked into these rooms for a long time and just sat down and I listened. I was hearing stories of other recovering addicts having the life I wanted. After showing up to weekly, sometimes daily, meetings, reaching out, getting a sponsor and working the 12 Steps, I have my Big Life: a life of connection with people of stability, trust, and not only liking myself but loving myself and the person I've become.

Final thought: Today. I am grateful to be an addict because I have learned the life skills I never had and could have learned only in MA.

April 7

Taking Inventory

"Through the process of taking inventory, we gain insight into our actions. We learn to recognize our motives and avoid rationalizing, minimizing, or justifying our behavior."

- Life with Hope, third edition, page 48

What made me so close-minded? Why did I have so many resentments? Maybe it was my marijuana addiction. When I started taking inventory of my life, I was amazed to discover that I had played a role in many of the situations and relationships that I was still harboring resentments and fears about. Smoking marijuana had dulled my self-awareness and made blaming others and running away from life easier. When I was actively using marijuana, not only was I powerless over my frequency of use, but I was also increasingly powerless over my emotions and reactions.

As I stayed clean for a while, I started gaining some self-control over these things. If I were to put marijuana to my mouth, that powerlessness would quickly return. The insights into my motives and behaviors that I gain from taking inventory of my life have resulted in emotional and spiritual growth. This growth enables me to stay clean, deal with life on life's terms, and even help others by sharing my experience, strength, and hope.

Final thought: Today, I will take inventory of my motives and admit when I am rationalizing, minimizing, or justifying my behavior.

April 8

Love Yourself First

"The joy of my life today is awareness of the details of life and in having the honesty not to want to change them."

- *Sharing Our Experience, Strength, and Hope: Personal Stories of Marijuana Addicts,*
MA pamphlet

I felt a lot of shame and guilt when I was smoking marijuana. I was ashamed of hurting the people that I loved. I felt guilty that I was unable to pursue my goals because I was high. I tried to hide the negative feelings that I had about myself. I was full of loneliness and despair.

In MA meetings, I heard people say, "you can't love someone else until you love yourself." As I worked the Steps with my sponsor, I realized that loving myself was essential to stopping my past destructive behaviors. My negative self-esteem influenced my desire to escape my feelings with marijuana. My sponsor told me that these feelings can also trigger a relapse if they persist. By doing the Steps suggested in MA, I learned how to positively build my self-esteem and my belief in myself. I asked my Higher Power to help me with my recovery; I knew that I couldn't recover by myself.

With recovery, I have learned that I am OK just the way I am. My Higher Power has unconditional love for me and this love brings me serenity and fulfillment. I want to improve my conscious contact with my Higher Power, so prayer and meditation have become part of my daily routine. I read a daily meditation every morning and I give thanks to my Higher Power every day.

Final thought: Today, my Higher Power leads me to a life of love; loneliness and isolation are no longer a part of my life.

April 9

Higher Power's Care

"Made a decision to turn our will and our lives over to the care of God, as we understood God."

- Life with Hope, second edition, page 11

Early in my recovery, I remember an MA member talking about Step Three, and pointing out that we don't turn our will and our lives over to a Higher Power, we turn it over to the care of a Higher Power. I grew up with the concept of a Higher Power that was judgmental and aloof. I certainly didn't feel that my Higher Power cared for me.

Fortunately for me, I also heard early in my recovery that I could fire my old idea of God, and create my own concept. I wasn't sure how to do this, but I was encouraged to act as if I had a Higher Power and that's what I did. To start praying, I recited the prayers I learned in recovery rooms. One day, I got the gift of feeling that there was a presence that cared about me. It was the first time in my life I didn't feel alone. It was a fabulous feeling, and I knew that if I used, I would lose it. This helped me stay clean in my first year.

I knew I wanted a Higher Power who was kind, comforting and non-judgmental. I don't have to ask my Higher Power for forgiveness because I am never judged. Eventually, I realized that faith means trusting I have a Higher Power, even though I can't see or touch it, or really know what it is. I have faith that I'm being cared for, and the proof is in the fact that I have been clean for half my life.

Final thought: Today, I turn my will and my life over to my Higher Power's care.

April 10

Rigorous Honesty

"Step One is about honesty, about giving up our delusions and coming to grips with reality. We had to look honestly at our relationship with marijuana and its effect on our lives."

- Life with Hope, third edition, page 3

Each time I smoked weed, my anxiety skyrocketed. Initially, I blamed it on my mood before smoking, thinking that a better mindset would lead to a different experience. However, even when I smoked in a positive state, I continued to feel intense anxiety and paranoia. My therapist, aware of my marijuana use, once asked if I thought I had a problem. I had always denied it, insisting that marijuana wasn't an issue for me. But this time, I broke down in tears and admitted, yes, it was a problem.

In the first four meetings, I struggled to openly admit to strangers that I was addicted to marijuana. It felt awkward and shameful, making me feel weak and vulnerable. I had always believed I was different, somehow above being an addict, so accepting that truth was a difficult realization. Hearing the Twelve Questions, I found myself answering yes to each one, realizing I was in the right place.

I've started sharing about my sobriety with close friends, which keeps me accountable and helps me actively practice Step One. I'm taking life one day at a time and am enjoying getting to know the person I am today. My former identity—seeing myself and being seen by others as a wife, baker, and pot dealer—is evolving into someone focused on becoming healthier and more self-actualized. My journey will always include God by my side, and sometimes carrying me through the tough times. I have faith that I'm on the path to a life beyond my wildest dreams!

Final thought: Today, I practice rigorous honesty, opening up my heart and mind and having the willingness to go to any lengths to have a spiritual awakening.

April 11

The Fourth Step

"Within the fellowship, we found that many of us had done the same kind of things, had felt the same, and had experienced similar thoughts."

- Life with Hope, first edition, page 17

"Look for the similarities, not the differences." When I first heard this, I found it hard to believe that this group of people were going to help me solve my overwhelming problems. I didn't trust myself, didn't trust anyone else and I was used to lying every day. Mostly to myself, but yes, my loved ones and employers got their weekly share of excuses and fabricated half-truths.

By the time I got to my Fourth Step, I had heard enough stories to realize that I wasn't "terminally unique." I had even laughed a time or two at the same convoluted thinking that had gotten my fellow stoners into trouble. Yes, I alternated between blaming myself and blaming others, but I really couldn't imagine another way of getting through life and its confusing unpredictable ways. I stopped trying to figure it out and just did it; promptly, with prayer and hope that it would bring some relief. Oddly enough, it did. I was scared and embarrassed but now I look at it as a list of things I might not have to do: lie, steal, cheat, or hang out with people who are not good for me just to stay high.

Final thought: Today, I can believe that honesty can be "more joyful than difficult" because I can better recognize the difference.

April 12

Acceptance is the Key

"Faith and acceptance are our new solutions."

- *Life With Hope*, first edition, page 13

This is one of my personal mantras. Everything starts from here. As with the Serenity Prayer, "God, grant me the serenity to <u>accept</u>..." When I get frustrated with anything, I stop and remember what is real. When I do that, then I can know how and where to move: forward, backward, or do nothing at all. I accept where I am, what is happening, and decide what can be done.

Final thought: With acceptance, I live in the present, not what was, or what could be, but what is; here and now.

April 13

Freedom from Resentment is My Key to Happiness

"After we listed and analyzed our resentments, we began to realize that they no longer had as much power over us."

- Life with Hope, first edition, page 19

I hold on to resentment like an old worn-out toy that no longer works. On the day of my 18-month recovery date, my house was full of people and activity not centered on me. I took my chip that evening hurt and angry, resenting that not one person in my home even knew about my 18-month chip. My resentment grew, as did my anger.

Leaving the meeting I recognized what a negative place my stinking thinking had taken me to. How did I know to reach for the tools of recovery? I just did; that's the miracle of recovery when I keep coming back. So, with willingness, and relief, in turning my resentment/anger over, I stopped at the market, bought a cake, entered my house with a smile, and invited everyone to join in my celebration.

Final thought: Today, I will turn over the thinking that gets in my way and become open to the joy of today.

April 14

Acceptance = Serenity

"We became responsible for our recovery and for letting God work within us."

- *Life With Hope*, first edition, page 25

Recovery has to be the priority in my life today, if I want a life worth living. It is not what happens to me, but how I respond to it, that determines my emotional well-being. When I was using, the smallest thing could set me off. I was filled with anger and resentment because the world seemed so unjust.

After I got clean, the anger, resentment, and fear were intensified. I could find no relief until I could accept that almost all of the things that happen to me are outside my control. I can control myself and my reactions to the world. When I choose to respond with fear and anger, I give people and events power over me and my emotional well-being suffers.

However, when I choose to accept the things I cannot change, and instead work on improving myself, when I ask for my Higher Power's help to respond in a positive way and to be of use to others, I find that the world is not such a bad place. I am able to feel better about myself and my place in the world. My spiritual and emotional well-being is enhanced and I am open to the possibility of serenity.

Final thought: Today, I will not let outside people or events control my emotional reactions.

April 15

The Fourth Step: A Writing Exercise

"The Twelve Steps of Marijuana Anonymous are to be lived, not just discussed in meetings."

- Life with Hope, second edition, page 43

When I first approached the Fourth Step, I spent much time talking about it, but little time actually writing. I took a piece of paper and wrote, "This is my Fourth Step" at the top and then promptly put the paper away. I sure talked a good game at meetings, but I did not work the Step.

Finally, my defects caused enough pain and I was able to work this Step. The majority of my work on the Fourth Step occurred on a long Saturday afternoon when I just wrote and wrote. I did additional work on it. I looked at my resentments, my fears and my sexual conduct. I put pen to paper. I had to keep reminding myself that this was my inventory, NOT the other person's!

It was hard work and brought up many feelings and reminded me of things I had forgotten. I was as fearless and thorough as possible. Soon after I took the Fifth Step with my sponsor, the closeness to Higher Power I felt at that point was beyond belief.

Final thought: Today, I will actively work the Steps, and not just talk about them at a meeting!

April 16

The Gift of Humility

"Our complete surrender and a new way of life were essential to our recovery."

- *Life With Hope*, first edition, page 4

When I first came into MA, I was doing pretty well in another 12-Step program. The MA meeting was small and my friends had asked me to help support the group, since they knew I had a history of using pot. As I sat in the rooms I felt a little smug because when I quit drinking I had held onto my baggie of "the good stuff" until I could find someone to appreciate it. I felt no urge to use and had totally forgotten how weed had ruled my life for years. Denial is an amazing thing. I had forgotten how I had driven miles to a sketchy neighborhood to score; how I had tossed away my college education to become a dealer. I had been in several situations that could have easily become felonies. It was illegal but I felt smug about the money; no fear, no humility, no sense.

As people shared, it brought back the memories of self-loathing that came when I couldn't make it to a family function; the shame of being high at work and hoping no one would notice; the inability to look someone in the eye; the lying, the nausea when the pot turned on me and stopped helping with the hangovers. When I heard a young boy about 11 saying his brother, the addict, got cranky when he wasn't high, it lifted my veils of denial. I knew if I ever had a joint in my hand I would definitely come to the day when I had booze in the other. My smug denial crashed, and I got grateful for MA.

Final thought: Today, I am grateful that I don't have to accidentally "lower my inhibitions" which keeps my "bottom" from getting any lower.

April 17

Removing the Eclipse from My Higher Power

"Although many of us came to the fellowship already believing in the existence of a Higher Power, we doubted that it would be of help since it had not helped us to stay clean before."

- Life with Hope, second edition, page 8

I had a Higher Power dating back to childhood, but it never helped me stay sober for long. There was a major flaw in my old relationship with this force. My lifelong concept of a Higher Power had a transcendent foundation in love, reality, and immutable laws of cause and effect. However, this was eclipsed by actions stemming from unexamined beliefs. I assumed my Higher Power was like an executive locked away from me in a top floor suite, disinterested unless I was far greater than all my human competition.

I had little acceptance or love of the present moment, as I believed only severe self-discipline and guile would gain me a promotion that would mainly come after death. I was to blame for my suffering because I had not manifested properly through my own thinking or metaphysical willpower. I had to be clever to unlock the gates of happiness. I needed the perfect balance of caffeine and THC.

In retrospect I have to say, that was a lot of pressure to put on myself. I treated life like it was an escape room! No wonder I made escapism my Higher Power. To begin my recovery, I had to separate my own precious plans for perfection from the Higher Power that could restore me to sanity.

Final thought: Today, I will reflect on the difference between my scheming intellect and a power greater than myself. I will do the best I can in all my actions, but then let mother nature do the rest.

April 18

The Greatest Adventure

"The story of Odysseus is about more than just a Greek guy in a boat. It's about the journey people take through life and the obstacles they meet along the way...As addicts, we were stuck in a Lotus Land; we forgot our mission; we forgot the other adventures that awaited us; we forgot about going home."

- The Story of the Lotus Eaters, *Life With Hope*, second edition, page xx

I find MA's literature so warm and cuddly. I love the story of The Lotus Eaters. When I first read this bonkers little bit of storytelling, I knew I was in the right fellowship. Reading it, I imagined an animated cartoon of the story. I love how MA encourages me to be creative and fun in my interpretation of its profound and deep messages. I particularly appreciate the subtle ambiguity in this story.

We never learn if the natives in Lotus Land are truly native to the island, or if they are other shipwrecked people who became hypnotized by the Lotus. There might be people for whom sitting around on an island, doing nothing but being lazy and eating lotus, is truly the best thing they can achieve in life.

I know that for me, despite spending nearly 20 years stoned out of my gourd every day, I am not a native of Lotus Land. I do have greater adventures in store for me, and a sincere calling to return to my true home. For me, I'm grateful that my inner Odysseus dragged me off the island. I'm so grateful for the adventures that I've had since that time.

Final thought: Today, I remind myself that I am the hero of my own story. The greatest adventure is what lies ahead. I continue to row like hell, remember my true home, and look forward to another adventure.

April 19

Honesty and Kindness

"Step One is about honesty, about giving up our delusions and coming to grips with reality. We had to look honestly at our relationship with marijuana and its effect on our lives."

- Life with Hope, third edition, page 3

It took me a long time to admit I was a marijuana addict. I had smoked dope almost daily all through my twenties. In my thirties and forties, though, I went through significant periods of time, even years, without smoking. I convinced myself that there wasn't a problem; however, I always found my way back to my old friend, marijuana. As marijuana started to become legal, it became all too easy for me to access it. One day, by grace, it dawned on me that I was an addict.

I have experience with other addictions and other 12-Step programs so I knew what to do. I went online and found my first MA meeting. I was immediately amazed at how much at home I felt there. It was as if I had found my people. I am 51 and have been without marijuana and in recovery for more than six months now. With the help of the 12 Steps, meetings, meditation and prayer, I work to stay vigilant, especially regarding my emotional sobriety and spiritual connectedness.

I will always be an addict and the dangers of cross-addiction are real, thus I have to stay honest with myself. Honesty means that I look at my thoughts and behavior with kindness and acceptance. I look at what I need to let go of and what I need to change. I believe that the slogan, "progress not perfection," has really helped me to accept myself and grow in recovery. Life is so much better living in alignment with my Higher Power and my own values.

Final thought: Today, I look at my thoughts and behaviors with honesty and kindness.

April 20

Willing To Be Willing

"There are many spiritual principles... honestly, openness, willingness..."

- Life With Hope, third edition, page 35

It is the phrase "willing to go any lengths" that sometimes makes me smile when I think back to my first meeting. I was desperate and had gone to the meeting location on two different days, but couldn't quite get out of the car. I had friends that had gotten clean and I knew that you asked someone to be your sponsor to help you get through the Steps in the book. I was doubtful, resistant and scared, but more frightened of going back to using.

I got out of the car, marched up to the nearest woman standing on those steps of the church, and asked her to be my temporary sponsor. She asked me if I was staying clean temporarily. Next, she asked me if I was willing to go to any lengths. I thought about those two questions the entire hour; I could barely hear the shares. I was willing to try, one day at a time. God knew the kind of sponsor I needed. I think of those questions and, sometimes, there comes a miracle.

Final thought: Today, I can be willing to be willing.

April 21

Not Just Existing, Living!

"I was existing—not living—from day to day in depression, not going anywhere or accomplishing anything."

- Growing Pains, *Life with Hope,* second edition, page 158

I remember doing homework in the common room of my freshman dorm, listening as two acquaintances talked about a short film they were preparing to shoot. As an aspiring actor, this made me angry; the guy who was going to direct the film knew that I acted, and he hadn't even bothered to tell me about it! He told the guy who was going to act for him, "don't show up high." It took me months of frustration and anxiety about why I wasn't picked to realize that I wasn't told about this project because, "don't show up high" was a demand I wouldn't have even understood!

This has been the biggest gift the program has given me; the feeling that I am not just existing, but living, too. I have strongly reconnected with my passion for acting and gotten to be involved in multiple theatre and film projects since finding Marijuana Anonymous. Those projects never would have been available to me had I not decided to get clean. When I was using, my dorm room was my home. I sat around smoking, playing video games, feeling lonely and sorry for myself.

This quote describes my life perfectly when I was using, and my life in recovery could not be more different. With medication and therapy, I have found ways to cope with anxiety and depression. Thanks to the program, I now have places to go and tasks to accomplish, too. I have learned how to live again, not just exist. I feel like I have a life that is worth living.

Final thought: Today, I will do one thing I can be proud of, because I remember what it felt like to have nothing to do.

April 22

Progress Not Perfection

"Just as denial once stopped us from seeking recovery, defiance, shame, and fear can hinder our spiritual growth."

- Life With Hope, first edition, page 15

I have been blessed with many years of clean time and I thank my Higher Power every day for getting that moment of clarity. I know that if I use any of my previous ways of coping, this beautiful life I get to experience will disappear and I'll be back in that pit of despair. This doesn't mean that every day is sheer delight, that everyone "gets" me all the time and that I don't have struggles.

Sometimes the biggest struggle is with myself. My defiance kicks in and I regress to a two-year-old having a tantrum or a sulking teenager who doesn't want to take out the trash or take care of myself. Sometimes I am riddled with shame because I intentionally used a cutting tone or remark to someone I love, or tried to get away with something that I know won't make me the person I want to be; the person with dignity because of my recovery. Some days, I have an obsessive fear over an unpaid bill or unresolved family situation, and serenity seems unobtainable.

That's when I pray, talk to another addict, plan for a meeting, and try to get some perspective. Recovery isn't a magic wand that makes my problems instantly vanish (which was what I was hoping for with pot). Recovery is a process with a lot of "baby steps." When I put my head on my pillow with another clean day, perhaps tomorrow will reveal a solution.

Final thought: I can "let go and let God" with practice and patience.

April 23

Learning to Say Yes

"It is not necessary to acquire a major God Consciousness to cease using. All we need is to maintain an open mind and a hopeful heart. It is not necessary to say yes. It is, however, important to stop saying no."

- Life with Hope, third edition, page 8

When I came into the program, I thought I understood God pretty well. I was the other side of the coin to those atheists, so sure there was no God. I didn't know how much alike we were, both sides so convinced we had the truth; end of discussion. It didn't end there; I wasted a lot of words trying to convince the other side that I was right.

In recovery, I've become agnostic—in the best sense of the word. I've gained a humility I never thought possible and when the convinced atheist arrives in our fellowship these days, I just shrug. I never get answers to ultimate questions; I get transformed by them. When I open my heart to wonder before the majestic miracle of my universe, marvel at the intelligence of ants with brains smaller than a grain of sand, stand awestruck under the night sky of stars and galaxies spinning out of sight infinitely, it's hard to believe anyone could possibly have "the answer," or the words to express it.

This doesn't make what I see, experience and feel any less real because it can't fit into a rational framework. It just points out the limits of my language and rational framework before the great mystery of life. What is important about that mystery is not that I understand it or express it or even that I experience it. What is crucial, at a minimum, is that I quit clenching my heart on my denial, and open myself, at last, to that wonder all around me.

Final thought: Today, I will quit saying "no" and I will practice opening my heart and mind to the wonders of life.

April 24

Shifting My Identity

"Going beyond our own self-interest and becoming concerned with the feelings and well being of others was new behavior."

- Life With Hope, second edition, page 28

My whole life revolved around pot—how to get it, where to get it, how to avoid getting busted, hiding it from my parents. I was a stoner, a pothead, a burnout. My use was my identity. Today, thanks to my recovery, I am so much more than those things. A part of me will always resonate with that identity, as that is what ties me to Marijuana Anonymous.

As I have progressed through this program and worked the Steps, I have been able to explore parts of myself that my smoking had diminished. I am still philosophical and laid-back, but now I am much more caring and present. I am much more connected to myself and those around me. I am good enough without the weed.

Final thought: Today, I value my identity as someone in recovery and embrace all aspects of myself.

April 25

Peace and Serenity

"We began to see the possibility that our beliefs about ourselves, formed while using, had been mistaken. We saw that our perceptions had been based in delusion."

- Life with Hope, first edition, page 6

I started smoking pot because I was uncomfortable and unhappy. I kept on doing it long after it started making me feel worse because I thought that unhappiness was my lot in life. I thought I was doing life wrong; I didn't have what it took to be happy, successful and loved. My life just was not going to work out.

I came to Marijuana Anonymous thinking I just needed to quit smoking and everything would be fine. Because I stuck around, got involved, got honest, took the suggestions, and worked the Steps, I was able to accept myself as I am; a person with a disease, doing the best I could with what I had.

I also got a new goal; not the "happiness" of ego gratification and getting what I want, but the peace, serenity, and freedom of living life on life's terms, clean and sober, one day at a time. Most of all, I learned that I am OK, and I am loved. I belong in the human race just as I am, and it is actually possible for me to be happy, joyous, and free.

Final thought: Today, I know that peace and serenity are available to me, so long as I stay clean and keep practicing these principles in all my affairs.

April 26

The Privilege of Having This Program

"The concept of one addict helping another and the privilege of practicing the Twelve Steps are very special gifts to marijuana addicts. The fact is that for thousands of years drug addicts and alcoholics had little or no hope of arresting their disease. For centuries upon centuries the disease was recognized, including the fact that it was sometimes familial. The Greek essayist Plutarch (born 46 A.D.) noted nearly two thousand years ago that, 'Drunkards beget drunkards.'"

- Working The Program, MA pamphlet

To me, it's incredible that for nearly as long as there has been the species *Homo sapiens*, there has been addiction. This fact does not usually make it into the history books. I cannot fully imagine what that must have been like for the loved ones and acquaintances of the addict. It sounds like that when one was identified as an addict, that person was likely considered a hopeless case. It feels like the greatest privilege is to be born in a time in which there is something called "recovery."

For myself, as recently as five years ago, I thought of myself as a hopeless case. I didn't know about a 12-Step program for marijuana. I was embarrassed. I didn't even think a person could be a marijuana addict. Early on in my recovery, I still felt embarrassed admitting in front of other addicts that my problem substance was marijuana. In fighting back against notions about marijuana being this evil substance, perhaps the pendulum swung too far in the opposite direction. Suddenly, everyone started treating marijuana as something harmless. I remember admitting my problem to old friends later on and them remarking, "Wow, I didn't even think you could get addicted to pot!" My addiction nearly drove me to extinction. I made regular promises to quit tomorrow, but I never could. Now, by practicing these principles, unavailable to many for thousands of years, a word like "fortunate" does not come close to how I feel.

Final thought: Today, I'm thoroughly unafraid to admit that I am powerless over marijuana. With this admission I feel powerful! I feel liberated!

April 27

Beginner's Mind and Continual Step Work

"Here are the steps we take which are suggested for recovery."

- How it Works, *Life with Hope*, third edition, page 193

There are very subtle aspects of Marijuana Anonymous' literature which I appreciate so much. Saying that these are the Steps we "take" rather than "took" is a seemingly small change from the way other fellowships have been written, but the consequences on my recovery were huge. In MA, I never felt like I had to trod gingerly in some giant's too-huge-to-fill footsteps in the snow, always worrying if I would thoroughly follow the path.

Marijuana Anonymous' phrasing makes me feel like I can take these Steps over and over again like a circle, and I needed that ease and comfort in order to take them the first time around. I have found that MA's approach to the Steps is warm, inviting, and exciting. Now, I'm on my third time through the Steps, and I learn so much more every time!

Final thought: Today, I look forward to discovering some new aspects of the Steps, trying my best to always keep a beginner's mind!

April 28

Dopeless Hope Fiends

"I need to relate with other human beings who, like me, became hopelessly addicted to what most people say is a harmless, non-addictive herb. I need to hear how other hopeless dope fiends became dopeless hope fiends."

- Freedom to Be Me, *Life With Hope*, second edition, page 131

For much of my using, I was surrounded by people who smoked like I did. Near the end, when I wanted to quit, I was around people who didn't know how much I smoked, and didn't believe marijuana could be addictive. It was hard having people not take marijuana addiction seriously. Once I finally made it to the rooms of recovery, I heard stories from other addicts that were just like me. In fact, there were a few stories that showed me I hadn't hit the bottom that they did. I've also realized that not everyone gets addicted to pot.

After being restored to sanity, I realize I'm one of the lucky ones, because being an addict gave me the gift of the 12-Step program, and a fellowship of people working to make their lives better. Where once I was hopeless and didn't think I'd ever be able to quit, now I am a dopeless hope fiend in recovery.

Final thought: Today, I am grateful for the worldwide fellowship of Marijuana Anonymous and the life recovery has given me.

April 29

A New Perspective on Resentments

"...we no longer have to behave in a certain way because of a resentment we acquired years ago"

- *Life with Hope,* first edition, page 24

I didn't start using pot until I was in college; however, I didn't enter the 12-Step rooms until my late thirties. I had been a resentment machine ever since I could remember. I admired the idea of peace and freedom but my mind and heart were filled with resentment. I resented that I was given up for adoption. I resented that my adoptive dad was a drunk and my mom would just go along with his outrageous behavior. I became resentful that college was getting in the way of my staying high. I resented that my boss expected me to show up for work on time, that my friends grew annoyed when I neglected plans and I became unreliable.

My massive ego and victim-stance made me miserable for years, but when I first got high I stopped caring and the resentment machine was silent for a bit. This was the answer to my problems. I resented that I couldn't stop using and resented people who could stop and those that had no interest in using. I had one goal, to stay high. I was sad and depressed over what my life had become but couldn't imagine a life without pot.

I made it into the rooms and worked the Steps. It took awhile but I could find moments of peace. I wasn't doing the stupid dishes, I was just cleaning up. That car wasn't cutting me off, it was just a careless driver. Sometimes, I get surprised by my own serenity; it's available if I work for it. I recognize what a gift 24 hours can be.

Final thought: Today, God is doing for me what I could never do for myself.

April 30

What's Passed is Past

"The pain of doing the Fourth Step was a lot less than the pain we would have held on to by not doing this step."

- *Life With Hope,* second edition, page 20

STEP FOUR, on the floor
Can't breathe, tears stream
So scared, prayer for care.
Addict mind, patterns I'll find,
Willingness, will it become forgiveness?
Resentful grudge, my soul's dark sludge
Scoff at humanity, in both you and me
Survival mode, the gaping God-shaped hole.
Fearless inventory, lend me some humility
Truly seeing clearly, seeking to be free.
Shedding my remorse, honest share with no recourse
Compassionate listening, will be oh so healing.
Rigorous honesty, if I'll ever get to know me.
Who's this sick lost child? Let me write a while...
Long-standing fear, still affecting me now and here
Ignorance isn't bliss, dissociate into the abyss.
What was my part? Courage in my heart,
Facing my selfishness, denial and bitterness,
Cheated and wrong, secrets held for too long
Not to criticize, but to realize.
World viewed in black-and-white; it's not 'wrong' or 'right.'
Can my character defect become a precious asset?
Can I give up control? Make readiness my goal
Shadows of my past, moving on at last.
Glad to be alive.

Final thought: Joyous and hopeful to step into FIVE!!

May 1

Step Five

"Speaking frankly about ourselves to our Higher Power and another human being expanded our self-knowledge, and relieved us of the burden of our past. A sense of belonging began to grow in us."

- Life with Hope, second edition, page 23

At first, the thought of taking my Fifth Step was terrifying. The idea of telling another person my deepest darkest secrets and revealing my soul was simply unimaginable; however, it was a necessary action to be taken immediately after completing my Fourth Step. Together, my sponsor and I took some deep breaths and said a prayer to invite my Higher Power. I began to relax enough to start reading my Fourth Step. As I spoke and she listened, the exact nature of my wrongs began to emerge. My behavior patterns and character defects clearly presented themselves. I was no longer terrified nor scared to face my true nature.

The amazing thing was that I no longer felt all alone and even began to feel like I belonged. I began to believe that my life was part of something bigger than myself. Sharing what I was so afraid to face with another human being actually changed my life. Learning to trust my Higher Power relieved my mind and provided a sense of belonging. I was now free to be myself for the first time in my life. My life began to get better, even beyond my wildest dreams.

During my addiction to marijuana and other mind-altering drugs, I had been so ashamed, embarrassed and uncomfortable in my own skin. I found peace, acceptance and relief in completing my Fifth Step. Now, I could move on with my Step work. I could grow up, be a productive member of society and even be happy, joyous, and free.

Final thought: Today, I wake up and ask, "How can I serve? What can I do for myself and others?" This is a far cry from the days when all that mattered was where I could find another joint.

May 2

Go Forth and Prosper

"By starting to trust our Higher Power, we cleared the way for growth and recovery."

- Life With Hope, second edition, page 13

After living a life as a marijuana addict, it is often hard to change one's life for the better. I have heard in meetings other addicts talk about all of the grandiose plans that were made while high, but never came to fruition. Lack of motivation and follow-through can often put life on pause. To make matters worse, the isolation and years of inactivity have made the very start of any worthwhile endeavor a painful and frightening experience.

Now, in recovery, I have been shown a path beyond a life of dreaming and procrastination. With the help of a power greater than myself, I can see that the only thing in my way is my own negative thoughts. If God is for me, who can be against me? This newfound motivation takes work and practice. The co-creative process of growth is not acquired by osmosis. I must learn that Higher Power works if I work with Higher Power, and therein lies the practice. Those dreams and aspirations I once had are attainable when I take the first step in their direction. Thinking about going back to school, writing a book, learning to play the piano, painting the next great American masterpiece is only a beginning. I also need to sign up for the class, call the piano teacher, grab pen and paper, and get those brushes and easel out of the closet.

I am built to be a demonstration of the awesome capabilities of my Higher Power. Fear, doubt, and worry are old emotions that no longer serve me. Recovery has taught me that together, my Higher Power and I can do anything. So I throw caution to the wind, rely on a power greater than myself, and walk hand-in-hand with Higher Power to accomplish my heartfelt goals.

Final thought: Today, I know I am capable of anything on which I set my sights. With Higher Power by my side, anything is possible.

May 3

The Objective Perspective of Step Five

"The inventory illuminated patterns of resentment, fear, and selfishness. We started to see their destructiveness. We realized, maybe for the first time, that these patterns were objectionable. Knowing this, we were free to act in new ways that made us happier and even brought joy to those around us."

- Life with Hope, second edition, page 22

Prior to Step Five, I was aware of the harmful quality of some of my thoughts and behaviors. They were objectionable, but I was unable to see them objectively. Sometimes I viewed this part of my life as one would perceive a garden that had become overrun with weeds. I would be overwhelmed and disgusted, thinking that I had hundreds of weeds that had become one massive, hopeless mess. I used avoidance and kept trying to start over in a new garden; yet the habits would follow to whatever new endeavor I began.

In Step Five my sponsor and I examined, row by row, my inventory. It quickly became clear that the problems I perpetuated could be narrowed down to a handful of common root causes, usually related to fear. I did not have hundreds of issues to address, nor did I have one unique, unsolvable dilemma. Through shining a light on the patterns of my character defects, I also began to realize that some of what I prized as the cash crops of my analogous garden were in fact liabilities, sowing misery. Steps Two and Three told me I didn't have to tend to this garden alone. In Step Five, with the help of my sponsor, I gained a hopeful, realistic perspective on my recovery landscape. There was still lots of work to do, but this Step provided a new objective view of the task list!

Final thought: Today, before taking any major action, I will pause to ask myself if the motivating factor is faith and service, or if by chance there are seeds of fear or selfishness. If I'm unsure, I'll bounce the idea off of a trusted third party.

May 4

Seeking

"Our Higher Power can and will if sought."

- How it Works, *Life With Hope*, third edition, page 193

One of the most beautiful ideas in Marijuana Anonymous is that my Higher Power can and will relieve my addiction "if sought." When I think about who I am in this spiritual journey, which is recovery, I think I am a searcher. This is a very good thing, since it is the search for my Higher Power that makes freedom from addiction possible. I came into MA looking for a way out of the hell of marijuana addiction. The people in this program showed me that there was a way, and if I keep searching for God, seeking the love and care of a Higher Power that is always there, I can live in freedom and serenity.

Final thought: Today, I will seek my Higher Power through working the Twelve Steps of Marijuana Anonymous.

May 5

Shortcomings Turned into Assets

"Within the fellowship, we can see and hear at virtually every meeting how people's lives of suffering have been transformed, by humility, into lives of happiness, fulfillment, and joy. Our greatest flaws and shortcomings can become our greatest assets in helping others recover from this disease."

- Life with Hope, first edition, pages 34-35

I believe that this is the main way my Higher Power works in my life. The things I didn't like about myself, my instincts taken to the extremes; the lying, cheating and stealing, are transformed into tools such as honesty. I can use honesty to connect with another pothead. It's the best part of the program. The newcomer can feel safe and brave to share experiences in meetings, with a sponsor and each other.

Final thought: A joy shared is multiplied, a sorrow shared is divided.

May 6

Our Primary Purpose

"We approach and make ourselves accessible to newcomers before and after meetings and during breaks."

- *Life With Hope*, second edition, page 64

In recovery, I have the opportunity to develop deep and lasting relationships with other people in the fellowship. Particularly in my home group I know the characters quite well, and can experience excitement at the familiar sight of them as I walk into the meeting room. However, it is always important to keep an eye out for unfamiliar faces and be ready to welcome new people, especially those who are new to recovery.

The Fifth Tradition of MA speaks directly to this principle, reminding me of my primary purpose to carry the message to the marijuana addict who still suffers. Meetings are often sprinkled with reminders to "keep coming back." I can encourage newcomers to keep coming back in many different ways. These can include briefly introducing myself personally before or after a meeting. It can include the ways in which I choose to share my stories, by being a living example of how a person can recover from the obsession of marijuana addiction by practicing spiritual principles with a mindset of progress not perfection. It can include sharing my phone number and following up with a call or text.

There is no minimum period of sobriety to make myself available to a newcomer. Those at every stage of recovery have something to offer. My existing friendships with others in recovery is important, but I must remain guarded against appearing as a member of an exclusive clique to newcomers.

Final thought: Today, I will think about a small step I can take to welcome a newcomer to MA.

May 7

The Dragons of Step Five

"This step helped us move towards sanity. It cut through our mental cobwebs like a sword and slew the dragons of delusion that had plagued us. We now find we no longer have to behave a certain way because of a resentment we acquired years ago. We no longer need to have the same kind of cavalier, selfish and manipulative attitude..."

- Life with Hope, first edition, page 24

I was so afraid of sharing with my sponsor what I had written in my inventory; I felt like hiding in the darkest corner, hoping it would go away. By this point in my recovery, I knew I had to face these dragons, these overwhelming fears and illusions keeping me from growing spiritually. After I had shared what I had written, I felt the shame and guilt that I had been carrying lift.

For the first time in years, I felt light, joyous, and free. The resentments and fears that had kept me toking for years no longer frightened me. I was now willing to face my life with a new design for living. No longer hiding from my problems, I acquired the spiritual tools that could actually relieve the burden one day at a time.

Final thought: Today, I will not fear the dragons of delusion. I will face today with eyes wide open and a willing heart.

May 8

If Nothing Changes, Nothing Changes

"Recovery from marijuana addiction requires us to make profound changes in how we live our lives."

- Life With Hope, third edition, page 41

When I came into recovery I just wanted to be able to stop smoking weed. The cravings were overwhelming and the temptations everywhere. It was suggested I change my patterns of with whom and where I spent my time. I stopped hanging out with my pot-smoking buddies and stopped frequenting bars and parties. I began to realize that my whole life had been shaped around my marijuana addiction. I had spent so much energy every day just trying to find it and get high.

My first sponsor said, "the only thing I had to change was everything." I got into recovery, started making new friends, and participating in new activities. As I continued working the program and doing service, I noticed my motivation and perceptions about myself changed. I began to practice new principles that were the opposite of my addictive behavior. I am amazed at all the time I now have and I'm glad to be part of Marijuana Anonymous. I am hardly the man I used to be, and I am becoming the man I always wanted to be!

Final thought: Today, I accept that change is inevitable and I embrace the new person inside me each and every day.

May 9

Spiritual Detoxification

"The Fifth Step can give a recovering addict a strong feeling of social connectedness and spiritual oneness....After all, it was heartening when we first discovered that actions which had filled us with shame and guilt could be understood and accepted by another person."

- Life with Hope, third edition, page 22

My Fourth and Fifth Steps were a spiritual detoxification. My sponsor gave the analogy of removing my guts to clean all the gunk around my organs before placing them gently back inside. As I procrastinated on my Fourth Step, I thought of my guts lying out on the floor, unable to return them until I shared with my sponsor. In the meantime, I had to stand there with my guts on the floor, exposed. My Higher Power called me to be thorough and honest, so I spent 40-50 hours writing my inventory. This much time is not required for everyone. I slept on the floor the last week until I was finished. This fast from my bed amplified the spiritual aspect.

When I finally shared my inventory with my sponsor, she listened for 11 hours with openness and acceptance. I felt vulnerable and raw. I never imagined someone identifying with the deepest, darkest corners of my being. Priding myself on acceptance of others, I felt shameful when I realized that one of my character defects was being judgmental—the root of many of my resentments. Not all sponsors do this, but mine helped me identify character defects and an amends list as I shared my inventory. That day I practiced humility, courage, and honesty. My sponsor practiced compassion and acceptance (and a ton of stamina). She helped me gather my guts off the floor and return them before sewing me up.

Together, we laid the groundwork to transform and overcome my defects. It turns out I'm not a bad person; I'm human. I can trust other people to accept me for who I am. I can also change. I've learned to rely on my Higher Power. I am worth loving; so are you.

Final thought: Today, I will experiment with vulnerability with at least one person and see what happens.

May 10

Trusting Our Higher Power

"Now we no longer have to rely on the weak force of self-will to solve our problems."

- Life With Hope, first edition, page 13

How freeing to read that it is arrogant to criticize myself! If I know that you're perfect just the way you are, how can I not believe the same about me? Am I suffering under the illusion of terminal uniqueness? Criticizing myself is just another form of self-centered fear. I came to recovery believing I needed to be perfect, and never make mistakes. In recovery, I've learned that's what humans do: make mistakes, and hopefully learn from them. As I learn to care for myself, and give myself the nurturing I've wanted from others, I feel freer, kinder, and more loving.

Final thought: Today, I accept myself the way I am, a perfectly imperfect child of the universe.

May 11

Unmanageability

"We admitted we were powerless over marijuana, that our lives had become unmanageable."

- Life With Hope, third edition, page 3

The unmanageability described in the First Step took me years to recognize, but eventually caused me enough pain to make me finally try to address my weed smoking and get clean. This is a two-part step. If I could smoke pot and live a manageable life, I would do it in a heartbeat. My experience shows me that as long as I am using, my life is unmanageable and always will be. Even if I could use just once a month, I would spend the rest of the month planning and fantasizing about what that one time would look like.

For me, it's just not worth it. I needed to be all out of excuses as to why my life was still working the way I had been living it. When I admitted that my life was unmanageable, I was finally ready to try sobriety. Although there is much more to sobriety and the MA way of life than staying clean, one day at a time, there are some days when staying clean is all I need to do for that day.

Final thought: Today, I give myself a chance to work the rest of the program, be of service and develop a relationship with a Higher Power. It works if you work it.

May 12

Let Go and Let God

"As we began recovering, we let go of convincing others what the Greater Power was, and instead focused on how to use that power in recovery."

- Life with Hope, second edition, page 9

One of the first slogans I clung to in early recovery was "let go and let God." I would say this to myself over and over while trying to learn how to meditate. Imagine my surprise, when after a couple decades of recovery, I realized that I rarely remember to "let God." I remember the "let go" often, but in truth I hardly ever really let go. How can my Higher Power help me if I cling to what is the current strife in my life? It can't. This realization brought me back to Step Two in a new way. Do I trust my Higher Power or not? I sometimes get so hung up on trying to define my Higher Power, I withhold my trust and faith.

I searched out recovery writings about faith and trust, and this helped me to truly begin to "let go and let God." What's been super helpful is the reminder that all I need to do is ASK. My Higher Power will step in, but not without an invitation; you know, free will and everything. I've also found it helpful to speak out loud to my Higher Power when asking for divine guidance. Please guide my thoughts and my actions.

Final thought: Today, I ask my Higher Power to guide me so that I can be of service to myself and others.

May 13

Facing Delusions

"This step helped us move toward sanity. It cut through our mental cobwebs like a sword and slew the dragons of delusions that plagued us. We now find we no longer have to behave a certain way because of a resentment we acquired years ago."

- Life With Hope, first edition, page 24

My active using compelled me to create a mask or false self. It was a story that I used to separate myself from my friends, family and co-workers. A secret paranoid fantasy of being the center of a plot in a spy novel, I would sneak around to continue to stay high, coming up with more and more ingenious methods for my subterfuge. I was the cosmic exception that proved the rule; however, I was just a powerless fool. Sharing my fears and resentments with my sponsor allowed me to see where these delusions had blocked me from an awakened authenticity in my relationships.

Final thought: I will share my delusions with a sponsor or trusted member, to help me to be the real me.

May 14

Willingness

"The form and timing of our amends varied according to the circumstances, but our attitude in each case was the same: willingness to take responsibility for the consequences of our behavior."

- *Life with Hope,* first edition, page 44

The Ninth Step is a series of actions I took in order to complete the work or process I began in Step Four: cleaning up the wreckage of my past. By the time I reached Step Nine, I had a good foundation for introspection, and was ready to take action. Step Nine is about accepting responsibility and cleaning up my side of the street. It is not done all at once. Sometimes donating to charity or working with others is all that is necessary.

Keeping in mind my side of the ledger is an important aspect of Step Nine. Empowered with an inventory of my resentments and fears, I could now go further and make amends to those whom I had caused suffering. Sometimes a simple apology was not possible, but it was always possible to make a living amends through right action. Donating time at institutions, sending out literature to the addict who still suffers, taking a service position in MA...are some examples of living amends. Turning it over and talking to my sponsor beforehand gave me the courage to face people I needed to speak with. I became a person of integrity.

Final thought: Today, I will remember that I can always make living amends by doing the right action.

May 15

Willing to Surrender

"Our inability to surrender had always blocked the effective entry of a Higher Power into our lives. Willingness was the lever with which we moved this obstruction."

- Life With Hope, first edition, page 11

My inability to surrender has brought me tears and frustration, particularly because I truly thought I had surrendered on numerous occasions. To surrender, I've learned, means to accept people, places, things, and situations as being exactly as they are at this moment. When I resist surrender, I create negative energy that blocks the spiritual connection between me and my Higher Power. The evidence of this blockage is that I become restless, irritable, and discontent. My character defects begin to appear and eventually take over.

In order to connect meaningfully on a daily basis with my Higher Power, I need to use my energy to practice willingness to surrender and accept life on life's terms instead of on my terms. Living life on my terms brings me depression, resentment, and relapse (with or without a substance). Living life on life's terms in harmony with my Higher Power brings me serenity, and I can then practice love and tolerance of others.

Final thought: Today, I will practice the willingness to accept things as they are right now, surrendering my will and my life to my Higher Power, using my energy to maintain the spiritual connection.

May 16

Being Happy, Joyous, and Free

"...lives of suffering have been transformed by humility, into lives of happiness, fulfillment, and joy."

- *Life with Hope,* first edition, page 34

When I entered recovery, I was extremely depressed and suicidal. There was nothing but sadness in my life and I could not see any alternative. I had suffered a lifetime of physical and mental abuse; I felt worthless and alone. From the time I was a child, I felt as though no one loved me. I was very shy and withdrawn and only spoke in a whisper. I lived in a fantasy world to escape my feelings.

When I took my first hit of marijuana, I was immediately transported; my cares were gone. Over time, I used marijuana as a method to escape. I became more withdrawn and isolated. I thought that it was helping my depression, not realizing that it was causing my depression to increase to the point that I became suicidal.

Being in recovery and working the Steps helped me cast aside these ingrained fears; having the love of a Higher Power gave me confidence. I learned to accept and love myself so that I could love others. Recovery has changed my life in so many ways and I am so grateful. The promises made in recovery have come true. Every day, I wake up grateful for another day of life in recovery. I count my many blessings. I have let go of my resentments and I have forgiven those who have caused me pain. I have let go of the painful, dysfunctional past. I give love freely. The inner peace that I feel radiates out to others. I find joy in my life every day.

Final thought: These days I am happy, joyous, and free! I feel gratitude for my recovery every day. Life is good; dreams come true!

May 17

Trust

"We did not fully trust ourselves, and trusted others even less."

- *Life With Hope*, second edition, page 21

Trust has been something I have had a hard time with my entire life. I never fully opened up to anyone and refused to actually let people into my world. When I was smoking, it made it that much harder to trust people. No one was allowed in my world because they could not be trusted with any information. It was only a matter of time before they would use that information against me. For many years, my lack of trust was paranoia from smoking marijuana, but once I finally quit, that paranoia lifted and trust became easier. When I started going to MA, not being able to trust was still with me, but once I finally started opening up with people in the rooms, it became easier to trust others outside of the rooms as well.

Final thought: Trust is hard, but a life without trust is harder.

May 18

Finding My Size

"We chose withdrawal and were egoistic, or we chose involvement and were self-effacing. On the one hand, we became so enamored with our own projects, plans, and personalities that we lost our humanity. On the other, we were so intensely involved in what others were doing that we lost ourselves."

- *Life with Hope,* third edition, page 26

I'm like many addicts I know whose ego is like a balloon with a slow leak. When I was active in my addiction, I always seemed to be occupied with inflating a deflating ego. I gave in to my deflation and threw myself into work, social, and political activism, or I chose a manic inflation that enabled me to fly away into my own empyrean isolation, and float high above the mortals below me. Eventually, I came to see that my ego inflation was as damaging to myself and my relations as my deflated self, and I looked around for anything that would dull the pain that damage caused.

For years cannabis was a temporary salve for the wounds, but eventually it ceased to have any impact at all. I now used it not because it worked, but because I couldn't stop. What had once been a solution now became just another wound in my ego. I realized I needed to deal with the wounds themselves if I hoped to have a "right-sized ego" and end my suffering.

I began to work the Steps, attend meetings, and do service in the program. I came back down to earth and began to build my life from the bottom up. Over time, I've reached an equilibrium and emotional balance I never before thought possible, and with that I've come to understand the meaning of the word, "serenity."

Final thought: Today, I will live my life in human community where I meet everyone as an equal and set the limits of my ego by that standard.

May 19

Working the Program

"We find that if we put top priority on spiritual growth, it is less likely that self-will and character defects will pull us down."

- Life With Hope, first edition, page 60

At an MA meeting one member spoke up and said, "If the train isn't moving there is no light at the end of the tunnel." He was talking about how we have to work the program daily to keep our sobriety. When I came into these rooms I wanted to get clean and experience serenity. In my experience, only when I got active, got a sponsor, and worked the Steps, did I have a spiritual awakening and a lasting sobriety, one day at a time.

I was told that I can't think myself into the right actions, I have to act my way into the right thinking, and the appropriate action is working the Steps. Faith is the key to open the door and board the Marijuana Anonymous Express. When I did, I was surrounded by commuters just like me on the way to a new life. I need to keep active in the program and get ready for what my Higher Power puts in my life.

My Higher Power is the conductor, my program is the train, and I am just a passenger. If the train isn't moving there's no light at the end of the tunnel.

Final thought: Today, I will get off the track of destruction, and ask my Higher Power to be the conductor!

May 20

Take it Easy and Take it as it Comes

"Our new attitudes bring about self-esteem, inner strength, and serenity that is not easily shaken by any of life's hard times."

- *Life with Hope,* first edition, page 68

The concepts of "easy does it" and "let go and let God" have been said in 12-Step programs for years and are well-known mottos. The concept of "taking it easy and taking it as it comes" combines those two ideas perfectly for me. When I think about "take it easy, take it as it comes," it reminds me that I am not in control of people, places, and things, like the car that won't let me into traffic, the individual that is not doing the things I think they should be doing, or whatever is bothering me at the time.

At my first meetings in the 12-Step rooms, I would see the mottos "easy does it," "one day at a time," and "let go and let God" on the walls and not really get it. Now, as I think of those mottos, I realize the great simplicity and depth of them. Thank goodness I did one other thing: kept coming back.

Final thought: Self-will and instincts are great survival skills, but I have to remind myself to take it easy and take it as it comes.

May 21

"Slowbriety"

"Marijuana Anonymous is a fellowship of people who share our experience, strength, and hope with each other that we may solve our common problem and help others to recover from marijuana addiction."

- Preamble, *Life With Hope*, third edition, page *xvii*

"Slowbriety" is not a real word—but maybe it should be. I took a long time to get sick and even to think about getting clean. If you were like me, you were getting high one day at a time thinking, "maybe tomorrow I'll get clean." Now, I'm staying clean one day at a time and rarely thinking I might get loaded tomorrow, but I know it could happen.

I have been in the program over 30 years and have slowly gotten better over time; slowly gotten better at dealing with life's difficulties and better at sharing about my successes. I have a lot more success the longer I stay clean and apply the program in my life. I hope I never lose my enthusiasm for recovery. There's a big difference in simply quitting getting high versus becoming a recovering addict and dealing with life's difficulties.

Final thought: Today, I will realize I am staying on the path of recovery and slowly getting better.

May 22

The Fifth Tradition

"Our primary purpose is to carry our message to the marijuana addict who still suffers."

- Life with Hope, second edition, page 82

When I first joined MA, I was badly in need of recovery, but there were many aspects of my life that were also sorely lacking. My spiritual and emotional life was a foreign, mostly unexplored landscape; but my social life was also in shambles, and my finances were a mess. As I grew along spiritual lines, I attended fellowship events like game nights, holiday parties, and social dinners after meetings. I became friends with members of the recovery community; I developed romantic feelings towards someone I met in the fellowship and I even entered into financial ventures with others who I grew to trust. These things were all well and good, so long as I remembered why I was there.

The Fifth Tradition reminds me that the primary purpose, the main reason I continue to go to meetings, is to carry our message to the suffering addict. In other words, the fellowship can serve many purposes, but the meetings themselves are not a social club. The meetings are not a dating pool. The meetings are not a business networking group. They are a place to do service and help newcomers.

As time passed, I developed stronger, healthier boundaries about how I interacted with people during meetings. I put aside my personal feelings towards people in the fellowship. I focused my shares on how to reach those who needed help. I made a concerted effort to welcome the newcomers, and to avoid cliques with friends. My actions have benefitted many newcomers and suffering addicts, but perhaps more importantly they've helped me to develop more spiritual integrity. Ultimately, this shelters me from the vicissitudes of my own biases and material desires.

Final thought: At each meeting, let me be of service by carrying the message to the suffering addict.

May 23

Freedom from Fear

"We began the journey toward becoming a true friend, a valued worker, a loving sibling, a trusted child, and a nurturing parent. We knew what our fears were and why we had them. They came out of the shadows and were a matter of record to ourselves, our sponsors or confidants, and to God."

- *Life With Hope*, second edition, page 24

Fear has been a major driving force in my life, and certainly while using. When I got high, I ran away from reality, hiding away from my fears about myself and the rest of the world. I figured if I was alone, then no one else could harm me or put expectations on me. I thought I was free, but I wasn't in charge; my addiction was. My fears of judgment, of rejection, of loneliness, all stemmed from my childhood and adolescent years. These formative years were very difficult and sometimes even traumatic for me. My teenagehood was spent feeling "less than" other people. I was afraid that I didn't deserve love unless I earned it. I felt that many people in my life seemed to demonstrate this as fact, including my father and my group of friends.

When I started working the program many years later, for the first time in my life, I was surrounded by a group that I felt truly cared about me and loved me for who I am. After that, I started to develop that same love for myself. I began to trust that I am good enough. I've done amazing things and proven to myself to be capable in many ways. I've found that when those fears come up now, they are often a source of growth and signal an opportunity to overcome that particular fear in order to become stronger. I listen to my Higher Power's wisdom and guidance, and I learn how to move through fear.

Final thought: Today, I look at fear as a compass I can use to find the direction Higher Power wants me to grow into. I take an action opposite to what that fear is telling me to do, in order to overcome it.

May 24

Suit Up and Show Up

"Then one of those nights hit when I ran out of pot. I was climbing the walls. I went crazy. I called everyone I knew to score even a roach. I remember one night driving 39 miles in a bad storm to get a half a joint from a complete stranger just to get through the night. I remember calling my dealer every hour on the hour to see if it had come in yet. I bought pot from people I normally wouldn't have even talked to much less done business with. What had happened to me? I thought I was using because I wanted to. Now I found that I was using because I had to. I had become an addict!"

- I'm Not an Addict, Life with Hope, second edition, page 147

For so long I did not want to believe I was a marijuana addict. I could not accept that I was powerless over marijuana. I remember sharing at a rehab that I would give up alcohol, and "drugs" but that I would never stop using marijuana. Needless to say, I did not get sober at that point. When I smoke marijuana it leads me right back to alcohol and other drugs. Yes, I'm a cross-addict! When I am smoking pot, I'm not living life! I don't want to work. I don't want to be social. I'm not there for my family, my friends, or anyone! I just want to live in my privately defined world, my couch, the TV, and a big bag of weed.

I am powerless over marijuana in all its forms. My life is not like that today. Most mornings when I wake up I feel good and ready to face my day, but when I don't, I get up anyway. I suit up and I show up. I am there for my family. I show up for work. I have many friends, especially sober friends. I enjoy life clean!

Final thought: Today, I will acknowledge my powerlessness. I will not use, and I will help another addict.

May 25

You Have Been Blessed, So Bless Others

"Luckily, we each had within us our own Odysseus, our own Higher Power, which grabbed us by the collar and threw us back into the boat. So now we're rowing like hell. We may not know what's going to come next, but we're back on our way through life again."

- Story of the Lotus Eaters, *Life With Hope*, first edition, page *xiv*

Being in recovery is like rowing a boat and not trying to steer it. I rely on the fact that when I try to steer, I go over the edge with expectations. I keep in my thoughts my gratitude and I am willing to row like hell. This helps me grow and look at myself today, and be able to look at my part. I realize that doing these simple things is all in God's time.

Final thought: Today, I will take my blessings with me and pass them on in a loving and caring way, relying on my Higher Power to steer the boat.

May 26

Acceptance, Courage, and Wisdom

"God, grant me the serenity to accept the things I cannot change, courage to change the things I can, and wisdom to know the difference."

- *Introduction to MA: A Meeting Format in a Pamphlet*, MA pamphlet

As a practicing pot addict, I was quite successful at getting nowhere fast. I was constantly moving mentally, which kept me one step ahead of my shadow. It was difficult for me to remain present emotionally because I was not processing my feelings and I was living in fear and denial. I had become comfortable being miserable. In early recovery, I found that the Serenity Prayer allowed me relief from my frayed being. It became my favorite tool. So easy, so immediate, was my respite. Its simplicity strengthened my resolve to move forward; one day at a time. It offers acceptance, courage, and wisdom. By becoming willing to bring a power greater than myself into my life, I was gaining more than I was giving up.

I cannot begin changing myself until I let go of the things I cannot change. For me, acceptance is a daily practice. Learning to feel and accept my feelings, good and bad alike, in real time affords me some perspective, some peace. Serenity begins to settle in as I slow down the internal dialogue. I calm down enough to summon my courage to start the hard work of actually changing the things I can. Attempting to change things beyond my control is exhausting and counterproductive. As I learn to distinguish the difference between what I can and cannot change, my daily outlook and attitude improves. Wisdom does, in fact, quietly sneak up on me when I practice honesty and service.

Final thought: Today, I will be aware of that which I have the power to change and keep it simple.

May 27

Restored to Wholeness

"Came to believe that a Power greater than ourselves could restore us to sanity."

- Life With Hope, first edition, page 5

When I first got clean and began working the Steps, I got stuck for quite awhile on the Second Step. Because I am an addict, because of actions I had taken in the past, the harm I had caused and my shame concerning those actions, I believed I was defective or broken in some way. I thought my insanity was how I had been created, that it was my basic nature.

Over time, I kept meditating on the words and meaning of the Second Step. I heard in a meeting one day that a key to this Step was the concept of restoration. I realized my healing as an addict was about restoration. I had not been created as a defective human, rather, I had experienced wounding and caused wounding in others. Indeed, the wounding I had caused others, also created wounding in myself. I was not broken or defective. I was wounded and had an opportunity for restorative healing.

My natural state is one of wholeness; within this wholeness is my healing potential. My Higher Power's limitlessness can restore any insanity, wounding, or imbalance in me. The compassion and gentleness of the availability of restoration is a healing balm for me. Over time, I have returned again and again to the idea of restoration. This opens a space of compassion for myself. It helps me have compassion for others who may have been, or might be, currently acting out of their wounds.

Final thought: Today, as I embrace the idea of restoration, I begin a healing process that helps me and my community. We heal.

May 28

Surrender to Win

"Gone were the days of insight. Now we experienced confusion, paranoia, and fear."

- Life with Hope, first edition, page 2

When I first started smoking cannabis, I got high, and I could laugh and see the world in a different light. A pocket full of cash and a pocket full of dope were my highest ambitions. However, within a matter of time, I became paranoid and constantly anxious. I could only get a bit of relief by smoking some more dope. It would only make me feel normal for about 30 minutes, then the hell of it all came back again. I was just using to feel normal, if only briefly. A tortured spirit, I had nowhere to turn but rehab and then to the support of other recovering addicts, and a loving power greater than me.

Final thought: Today, I don't have to be a tortured spirit. Today, I have hope, serenity, and fellowship of others in recovery. Today, I'm heading in the right direction.

May 29

Into Action

"Marijuana gave me wings to fly, and took away the sky."

- Freedom to Be Me, *Life With Hope*, third edition, page 116

The longer I am clean, the more I realize how much thinking I used to do. I spent hours daydreaming and creating imaginative plans in my head about all of the things I could do tomorrow. I put off my goals and dreams and instead I smoked away any real motivation I had left while dreaming up more plans. By the end of the day, I would be exhausted simply from all the thinking I'd been doing!

In MA, I have learned to focus on what I can do today. I have learned to get in touch with my goals and aspirations while consulting God for guidance. While I still have my imagination, I am now able to take action. I am able to put one foot in front of the other and walk a path of recovery one day at a time. When I fantasize about escaping through marijuana into the depths of my own mind, I can remember how much more I've been able to accomplish since I quit using. I now have a fellowship I can connect with and a Higher Power that I can rely on.

Final thought: God, help me remember today that I am much more capable of accomplishing my goals if I stay clean and rely on You. Help me put one foot in front of the other and take the next indicated action.

May 30

Cross Addiction

"We addicts have a dangerous tendency to self-medicate."

- Dangers of Cross Addiction, MA pamphlet

In recovery, I encounter many new people with lots of new ideas, and hear many stories about how to negotiate this new path. It can feel overwhelming and seem unattainable. I am offered many suggestions and loving support. I try to accept these gifts as I build momentum one day at a time. It is hard to let go of old patterns. Sometimes, I am subconsciously holding onto a marked card: a hidden urge to act out in some other way. These urges can end up surfacing later as flirtations with alcohol, overeating, use of other drugs or behaviors that are unhealthy. This is referred to as keeping one foot out the door.

My relapses on pot can happen as a response to family, work, or relationship issues that push me over my stress limits. Sadness, anger, fear, loneliness, or other emotions overcome me and I am unable or not willing to process the pain. As an addict, I have spent years fulfilling my desires with instant gratification but that is not a viable option now. When feelings push and pull me apart, my mental state is at risk. These triggers can sneak up on me before I am consciously aware of them. This is the time to call a friend or sponsor, take a walk or just attempt to feel the feelings, and let time work its magic. I do not have to suffer in isolation or punish myself.

Final thought: Today, I will feel my feelings and be aware of triggers that may sidetrack me.

May 31

The Reality of Powerlessness

"In Marijuana Anonymous we discover the reality of powerlessness; surrender outweighs the illusion of control and becomes our only option for recovery. We are powerless over marijuana in all of its forms."

- Life With Hope, third edition, page 4

I find it helpful to repeat the following to myself aloud daily while working Step One and beyond:

"I am completely powerless over marijuana. If I use, I am sure to do it again. I cannot control or moderate my marijuana use. It is imperative that I surrender my addiction to God and commit 100 percent to not using again, even once, or I will spiral out of control, as I have done so many times before. God's purpose for me is not to be merely functional, or be content with mediocrity. God's purpose is for me to reach my full potential and grow into a full-fledged butterfly, one step at a time. I surrender my delusion that I can use once in a while and still grow. To grow as God intends for me, I must surrender completely."

This is my foundation.

Final thought: Today, I will not use marijuana.

June 1

Transforming My Character Defects

"...Step Six was a step that required just as much, if not more, action. The action we took was becoming entirely ready to let our Higher Power remove or transform these imperfections of our character.

- *Life with Hope*, first edition, page 28

I am attached to my character defects. I hold grudges, and I enjoy holding grudges. I'm vain, and that makes me feel nice. I like to gossip, because it's fun. Why would I ever give these character defects up? The chapter in *Life with Hope* on Step Six talks about the ineffectiveness of our defects in managing our lives, versus the effectiveness of our virtues. Gossiping might be fun, but it only builds resentments that might cause me to relapse. Vanity might make me feel nice, but where does it get me? As to holding grudges, an unwillingness to forgive is a sickness unto itself.

These thoughts are easy to conceptualize, but how do I act on them? How do I become even slightly willing, much less entirely willing, to have my Higher Power as I understand it, remove these defects of character, when I enjoy them so much? Even if these defects aren't removed by my Higher Power, they might be transformed. Vanity can be diffused into self-care leading to self-worth, instead of self-pride. Instead of gossiping about someone, I can address my judgment-free comments, concerns, and opinions directly which would lead not to resentment, but constructive discussion. However, grudges must be entirely removed. They are a sickness as grave as addiction, and no action will transform them into forgiveness except the willingness to have them removed. These positive methods are far more effective in managing my life. It will take action on my part. Guided by my Higher Power, I manage my actions and reactions in these positive directions.

Final thought: Today, I will take action. Today, I will be willing to transform.

June 2

Our Biggest Treasure

"We say, 'we take' these Steps, not 'we took' them, because we live these Steps continually."

- *Working the Program*, MA pamphlet

The most treasured part of recovery to me, besides the fact that it has saved and transformed my life, is that the serenity I find is a daily reprieve. There is no day so awful that I cannot find a peaceful solution in the Steps; no action I can commit that is horrendous enough to take away the tools I have been given so freely. Every day, I can admit the powerlessness that leaves me stuck, understand that it is not up to me to fix it, and turn over my pain. I get to find the roots of my discomfort, confide in another about it, and then have them removed.

I clean my own house, connect to the Higher Power that helps me keep it clean, and spread the message of my continually-found peace; every single day. It is a gift beyond words to have the conscious daily opportunity to start over; to be able to surrender completely and continually to life on life's terms, armed with solutions to any and all of life's hardships in my Steps.

Final thought: Today, I collect my daily reprieve of serenity through continuously working the Steps.

June 3

Making that Connection

"Character defects are, by their very nature, expressions of self-will."

- Life with Hope, first edition, page 25

When I am acting in my character defects, when I am gossiping, when I am nasty, when I am unsympathetic or unkind (even when I've asked God to remove these same defects of character); it is often because I am unsatisfied in some way. When I closely examine that feeling of irritability, I am able to see how my will is misaligned with that of my Higher Power's.

Once I have that realization, my next step is to accept that which I am currently finding unacceptable. How do I do that? I turn to God for help. Even though I may not initially make the connection between my own bad behavior and my lack of comfort in a given situation, it is that very connection that must be made in order to rid myself of those character defects.

As soon as I'm able to see that connection, I need to ask God to direct my thinking and to help me to be of service. Oftentimes, as if by magic, I am able to not act on those defects. Going forward, if I remember to align my will with God's, I find that I do a better job in managing my character defects.

Final thought: Today, I ask God to help my will be aligned with my Higher Power's so I can be free of my character defects.

June 4

Accepting Feelings

"When we acknowledged and accepted our feelings, we behaved moderately. We ran less risk of relapsing or of switching addictions."

- Life With Hope, second edition, page 35

Before getting clean and working the Steps, I would do anything to avoid my feelings. I had become such an expert at avoidance that when I came into MA, I had to relearn how to feel, both recognizing what my emotions were and how to just sit with them. When I was using, I only wanted to get away from my feelings as quickly as possible. Since my addiction is a "disease of more," it sometimes led me to seek an enhancement in a moment of celebration. Most of the time, marijuana was a way to diminish and escape, especially what I considered the unpleasant emotions of anger, fear, and sadness.

In recovery, I have discovered that my emotions are a necessary part of being fully human. I have also learned that I can acknowledge, accept, and not overreact to any particular feeling, allowing each to arise and dissipate. Like everything else in life, feelings change, and I know now that I needn't be afraid of them, because they will always subside.

Final thought: Today, I do my best to acknowledge and accept my feelings.

June 5

Actions and Motivations

"The difference between our defects and our virtues is their effectiveness in helping us live clean, spiritual lives."

- Life with Hope, first edition, pages 27-28

I feel that in many ways Step Six is the action step related to Step Three. When I make a decision to turn my will and my life over to my Higher Power, that manifests itself in Step Six as a willingness to have my character defects removed. The problem is that it is not always so clear cut what is a defect and what is a virtue; for example, some amount of confidence may be necessary at work when I need to defend my work product, but if I am so prideful that I step on the opinions of my co-workers, my confidence has become a defect.

If I measure my actions and motivations by their effectiveness in helping me to live a clean spiritual life, it provides me with a clear benchmark to tell when I have crossed the line, so that next time, with willingness and humility as my guide, I can do something different.

Final thought: Today, I will seek the clarity to recognize when my actions are manifestations of my character defects and when they are moving me closer to my Higher Power's will for me.

June 6

Service Connects Us

"What we learned is that recovery from addiction requires resources beyond the capacity of any one individual addict."

- *Life With Hope*, third edition, page 9

I used marijuana in isolation. When I was with others for work or socially, I couldn't wait to get back home to smoke. I was impatient and not fully present with others or in what I was doing. Even with smoking friends, I preferred to use alone, at a high enough level to maintain the insulation from feelings. Isolating myself ever further from deep, meaningful relationships, I hid out in my garage alone.

Hearing the stories and feelings described by other addicts in meetings was the first time, in a long time, that I felt close to other human beings in a way that wasn't superficial. In my first weeks of sobriety, I attended between two and four meetings a day. Now, I still attend one or two meetings a day. I attend a book study group and online fellowship. I laugh and cry and call fellows. I feel empathy and compassion for others. I have service positions in several meetings.

Helping and being helped by other addicts, the fellowship is now doing for me what I could not do for myself. As I work the Steps, I am discovering the nearness and comfort of learning where I end and my Higher Power takes over. Only during this clean time have I felt the depth of God in the faces, voices, and words of my fellows. I am so grateful that Marijuana Anonymous is here for us.

Final thought: Today, I will attend an MA meeting to feel connected with other addicts, to be of service, and to grow in sobriety.

June 7

Freedom from Self-Obsession

"We learned that the more we could let go of our selfishness and try to carry out what we perceived as God's will, the more we started to experience serenity in our lives.

- Life with Hope, third edition, page 31

When I first came to MA and learned that selfishness is a common feature of addicts, I didn't think that trait applied to me. I always thought of myself as the kind of person who was there for friends and family when they needed help. As I began to look at my history of marijuana use, I started to see that I had prioritized getting high above many other parts of my life, including personal relationships, school, and work. Later in my recovery, as I wrote my Step Four fear inventory, I discovered I had a deep-seated fear of being selfish. In working Steps Six and Seven, I became willing to let the God of my understanding remove my fears.

As I continue to work the Steps and apply them in all aspects of my life, I am more aware of how often my thoughts veer towards self-obsession, which is a painful form of selfishness. I have found a solution to this problem: asking God to steer my life and my thoughts away from myself and towards others whom I can serve. When I become aware of obsessive and/or self-directed thinking, all I have to do is ask my Higher Power to remove these thoughts. I can then reach out to someone I can help, which can be as simple as making a phone call to a fellow addict. I have found that taking these small actions brings me true satisfaction and serenity. I've begun to understand that my true will is perfectly aligned with God's will for my life.

Final thought: Today God, help me to become aware of when my thoughts are self-directed and to ask for your guidance and support to turn my thoughts and actions toward someone I can help.

June 8

Freedom is a Real Possibility

"We are transformed from suffering addicts seeking relief from the grip of our disease into people who are able to be 'happy, joyous, and free.' By the grace of a Higher Power, we are given the gift of recovery."

- Life With Hope, third edition, page 57

By the time I made my way to Marijuana Anonymous, I must have attempted to quit...to be honest, I can't remember how many times I had attempted to quit. I know it's been many, many times. Each time I wound up one way or another with a pipe in my face, thinking to myself, "This is the last time," before taking a deep, deep inhale.

Little did I know that the day I attended my first Marijuana Anonymous meeting was the day my relationship with marijuana and, even more deeply, my relationship with myself would change forever. I never thought freedom was possible for someone like me. Could I have a life without the desire to get high, and even more mind-bogglingly, a clean life that is full of joy, mystery, and love? I know it now through my own direct experience that such radical personal transformation is possible and, because it's possible for me, I know it's possible for other suffering addicts as well. Freedom is a real possibility.

Final thought: Today, I live my life in awe of all the wonderful and mysterious experiences life has to offer. Today, I live my life with freedom.

June 9

A Newfound Awareness

"Character defects are, by their very nature, expressions of self-will. We realized that by practicing them it was impossible to practice spiritual principles."

- Life with Hope, first edition, page 25

I took the tack that was perhaps a dangerous and heartbreaking one; I was fatalistic. I accepted other people's constraints on my needs, desires, and ambitions. I believed that my lot in life was inevitable, inescapable, and miserable. Finally, I reached the point where my disease enslaved me and I was too stoned to know it. My needs were unfulfilled, my passions frustrated, and my ambitions thwarted because I could not see the forest through the trees. The sad fact was that I cruelly and piteously oppressed myself and usually found other people who were more than willing to help me do so.

By doing Step Six, my newfound awareness was making it impossible for me to comfortably continue practicing my character defects. Going beyond my own self-interest and becoming concerned with the feelings and well being of others was new behavior for me. This new attitude was contrary to my prior self-obsession, which had in fact been the root of my disease.

Final thought: Today, I practice recovery by being entirely ready to have God remove all my defects of character.

June 10

The Next Right Thing

"I was told that you can't think yourself into the right actions, you have to act your way into the right thinking..."

- My Best Thinking Got Me Here, *Life With Hope*, second edition, page 176

The phrase "fake it until you make it" sums up so much of my experience in recovery. Just because I got clean and sober doesn't mean that my disordered attitude, thoughts, or behavior have automatically been transformed. There are many days when I don't want to pray, I don't want to go to a meeting, and I don't want to check in with my sponsor or another fellow. There are moments when I find myself consumed by much of the same negative self-talk that drove me to escape with marijuana for so many years; however, my thoughts don't have to dictate my actions.

I have learned in recovery to pause, breathe, and do the next right thing. I try to act "as if" I am already the person I would like to be and trust that where my body goes, my mind will follow. I may not ever rid myself of my "stinking thinking," but I sure don't have to listen to it. Because of the fellowship, I can recognize my overwhelming feelings, accept them for what they are, and make more effective decisions for navigating them.

Final thought: Today, I will act "as if" I'm already the person I would like to be by doing the next right thing. When I am not sure what to do, I will lean on the fellowship.

June 11

Living with Faith

"Recovery...begins with a real desire to stop using, with a genuine change in our attitude, with a soul-transforming realization that we are finally willing to go to any lengths to change our lives."

- Life with Hope, second edition, page 4

Stepping into recovery rooms for the first time was terrifying. I knew it would no longer be possible to deny my addiction. I was there to admit it to others as well as to myself. I could grasp that I was powerless over marijuana but I had no idea what it meant to go to any lengths to change my life or what it would mean to have a spiritual awakening. The answers did not come immediately. I attended meetings regularly and listened as others shared how they had learned to live by spiritual principles and to seek support from a loving Higher Power to guide them to live "life on life's terms." My "attitude of gratitude" grew as the days passed. I started to believe that my life could be transformed from being angry and self-serving to being at peace and in service to my fellows. While it wasn't always obvious, I began to notice how I was living with faith, that every new day held promise instead of dread.

After some time, I got a sponsor and began working the Steps. I was willing to examine, define, and understand my past behaviors, to ask God to remove my character defects, and forgive myself and others. My willingness to turn my will over to God's care opened a path to see my life as having a positive purpose. I was proud to be living this life, having achieved the humility to recognize that I was living out God's will for me.

Final thought: Today, marks a new beginning as I surrender my will to a Higher Power and trust that, with its love and guidance, I will succeed in living life along spiritual lines.

June 12

Greater Power

"As we began recovering, we let go of convincing others what the Greater Power was, and instead focused on how to use that power in recovery."

- Life With Hope, third edition, page 10

When I entered recovery, I secretly wanted to share the God ideas I had from years of study. I liked the open-minded nature of the rooms, yet really wanted my God at the center somehow...or rather, for me to somehow be able to impart special healing wisdom from my learned perspective of God as love, life, truth, principle, soul, and spirit. Honestly, I still yearn to really understand, to feel this magnificent, ever present God and to share the light through me. As days and weeks and years go by, I find myself just needing to be cared for and heard unconditionally, on my path to recovery.

Final thought: Today, my Greater Power is acceptance of recovery in all its forms.

June 13

Present Moment Awareness

"Our mental life becomes focused more and more upon the here and now and less and less upon the past or future. Often, we can admit our mistakes as soon as we make them."

- Life with Hope, second edition, page 51

I noticed that after a few years of clean time, I have been able to continually develop my spiritual muscles. The daily spiritual practice of meditation and gratitude helps me focus more on the beauty of the present moment. Less and less do I regret my past or worry about my future. I am able to be more cognizant of when these feelings arise and I am able to nip the distressing feelings in the bud, leading to a more consistent state of peace and serenity.

From time to time, anxious thoughts do creep in, but I am able to witness the anxiety-ridden thoughts and the tense bodily sensations pulling at my heart. After this period of awareness, I simply label the situation as what it is, anxiety, stress, rumination, anger, or whatever it may be. By labeling it as nothing but intrusive thinking and my mind wandering away from the present, I immediately gain back my power and control. In addition, I utilize the healthy coping behaviors I learned through the program: call a friend, call my sponsor, meditate, deep breathe, and I "let go and let God," regaining my presence.

Final thought: Today, I focus on the here and now.

June 14

Grandiosity

"Were we full of tremendous insights, but unable to follow through with the vast projects we envisioned?"

- Life With Hope, first edition, page 17

Tremendous grandiosity and belly laughing was what started me down the path of smoking pot and living a life with passion. My mind was on fire with creativity. People hired me for unique fabric art and clothing. I gave most of the credit to being high, so it gave me a reason to smoke. I started missing deadlines and not completing projects. I didn't see the correlation. I just kept consuming, not knowing when it became an addiction until a friend confronted me.

I checked into treatment and learned that I was a drug addict and not picking up again could change my life—Step One. Shortly after graduation, I was in a serious car accident; and as an agnostic, I was shocked to hear myself say, "God help me"—Step Two. I hit my real bottom. I surrendered to moving in with my baby sister—Step Three—and started meditating—Step Eleven—to keep the pain at bay. I found my sponsor in my women's group and did what she said.

I started a crewel embroidery piece which gave me something to do with my hands and reignited my love of fabric—I learned to follow through. My second sponsor helped me really have a more open and honest program. Then, I found MA; I was home. I will admit that even today, I can have great ideas and not follow through, but it isn't as often because I finally have the life tools to complete the projects.

Final thought: Today, I will breathe deeply, quiet my mind and listen to my Higher Power's and the fellowship's guidance.

June 15

Self-Acceptance

"Many of us discovered that we had low self-esteem. We learned that we are neither all bad, nor all good. We are simply human."

- Life with Hope, third edition, page 19

When I was using marijuana, I had an artificial sense of self-acceptance. I thought that I was cruising through life with grace and had everything under control. It was only when I got clean that my lack of self-acceptance was unveiled. I didn't know who I was when I was not escaping from my problems and character defects. I was quick to judge my past mistakes and I held resentments towards myself for not seeing the negative impact I had on the people in my life. I thought I was the worst of the worst.

Once I began working on the Steps, I came to the realization that humans are imperfect, striving for progress, not perfection. All that matters is the willingness to right my wrongs and accept myself when things do not go to plan. I seek my Higher Power to help guide me through my day-to-day life. My self-esteem is based on esteemable acts in which I engage. I no longer have to carry the weight that I am "not good enough." I am simply human. I am clean, and that is more than enough.

Final thought: Today, my self-acceptance depends upon my willingness to do the next right thing, and to engage in esteemable acts.

June 16

Powerless Over My Marijuana Use

> "Until we admitted our powerlessness, denial kept us from realizing how unmanageable our lives had become."
>
> - *Life With Hope*, first edition, page 3

Admitting I was powerless was no easy task. Powerless, I thought, meant a sign of weakness, a step down, maybe even thoughts of being "less than." However, according to the text, I needed acceptance of my powerlessness in order to see how unmanageable my life had become. When I started working the Steps and looking at my marijuana usage, powerless soon began to take on a new meaning. Once I took the first hit of marijuana, I was powerless over when I took the next one. The need to smoke, the desire to smoke was out of my control. I was, in fact, powerless.

After a few months in recovery, thoughts of needing to give up, to surrender, to let go came to my mind when I thought of being powerless. The unmanageability aspect was not being able to manage my life; it was my inability to manage my usage once I smoked. Once I took a hit, I lost the ability to quit. I had to surrender and let go of any thoughts of controlling my usage.

Final thought: Today, I will remember that this decision to surrender, to accept defeat, was powerful and made it easier to see just how unmanageable my life became when, and/or if I smoked.

June 17

A Daily Practice

"As addicts, we were stuck in a Lotus Land; we forgot our mission; we forgot the other adventures that awaited us; we forgot about going home."

- The Story of the Lotus Eaters, Life with Hope, first edition, page xiv

The First Step included admitting our lives were unmanageable. As an addict, I have to try every day to release my desire to control. Every day is a practice of letting my Higher Power into my life. It's getting easier to distinguish my Higher Power's will from my own. Every day is a practice of humility. Every day is progress if I allow it. Every day I remind myself to be gentle. There are positive and negative energies all around me in recovery every day.

Final thought: Today, I will do my best to tap into the positive. I can start right now by counting my blessings.

June 18

The Fantasy of Functionality

"We were living the fantasy of functionality."

- Life With Hope, second edition, page 2

I'd traveled widely, learned a second language, and made friends around the world. A therapist suggested I go to 12-Step meetings. I debated her. After all, my life looked pretty good. I'd kept in good shape and I'd had some beautiful lovers. I'd produced a portfolio of creative work and I didn't owe a dollar to anyone. I was a strong student in a renowned doctoral program. Sure, I was high when I went to class and I was high when I wrote my papers, but I earned A's and had an impressive dissertation in the works. It was hardly a picture of addiction. I made that case for the better part of a year before I ran out of rope.

The truth was that I was far from satisfied. I knew my accomplishments weren't the result of disciplined effort and personal growth. I knew my relationships lacked rigorous honesty and genuine intimacy. Above all, I knew that I was constantly apprehensive, lonely, and sad. I had to accept that I was just skating by. Sure, some of my tricks scored points, but I didn't really care what the judges thought. There was no joy in my routine and the thin ice was cracking beneath me. I was terrified of the dark and frigid abyss that I imagined below; but I came to accept that if I was going to feel better, I was going to have to take the plunge. It was cold for quite awhile. I learned to accept that too, along with so many other things. Slowly, with the help of fellows, I swam to warmer waters. Eventually, I began to trudge the solid but uneven ground of life on life's terms.

Final thought: Today, that ground is the foundation of my serenity.

June 19

No Amount is OK for Me

"The truth is that I am a marijuana addict, and I will never again be able to smoke pot like a non-addicted human being...I don't have any brakes to slow me down."

- Started Off with a Bang, Life with Hope, third edition, page 113

I didn't have a hard time accepting I was an addict. After 25 years of consuming copious amounts of marijuana, many of those years on an hourly basis, with the exception of sleeping hours when I would only smoke every two to three hours, I knew I was an addict. The thing that I was reluctant to accept was that I wasn't ever going to be able to smoke weed like a "normal" human being. Any time I would manage to put together a few days or a couple weeks of sobriety, I would reward myself with a joint, have a few hits, and throw it away. This would be followed by a gradual increase in smoking marijuana. I hung tightly to the idea that I was capable of just smoking occasionally, or just on holidays, if I could just improve my self-control.

It wasn't until I accepted the idea that to stay clean meant that there would never be any weed in my future, that I found relief. No amount, regardless of how small or how infrequent, would be OK for me. It was OK for non-addicted people, but not for me. Once I let go of the idea that if I could fix my self-control or my willpower and then I would be able to smoke occasionally with control, my life changed drastically. I was one of the lucky ones whose desire to get stoned lifted immediately.

Final thought: Today, I accept that as an addicted person, no amount of weed will ever be OK, and no amount of self control will keep me from relapsing.

June 20

Living in the Moment

"...being aware of what we are saying, staying present...is a moving and powerful experience."

- *Life With Hope*, second edition, page 58

When I am living in the moment—not "future tripping," as they say—I am more acutely aware of my feelings. This always proves helpful in dealing with my crazy addict mind. When I am present, it is easier for me to fully embrace my place in God's universe and for me to accept that I am an agent of that force. In this awareness, I may be of better use to my fellows. I might actually stand a chance at being compassionate toward all, and most importantly for this addict, to tolerate that which I cannot understand. Being present can be as simple as taking, holding, and finally exhaling a breath. I am allowed to do this. I am allowed to do nothing but breathe and be, and come into awareness. I am allowed, in this manner, to take time out from my busy day and sit calmly with myself and thoroughly take stock of my desires, needs, and wants. When I am in such a state, I can more effectively weed out my crazy thoughts, so that I may come closer to doing God's will.

Final thought: For today, I will set aside a few moments to be keenly present, with the goal that I may be present throughout the day and aware of my feelings, desires, needs, and wants.

June 21

Daily Meditations

"Sought through prayer and meditation to improve our conscious contact with God..."

- *Life with Hope,* first edition, page 55

Recovery is a matter of life and death. Every moment of every day, I make the choice to stay awake to the essential truth of my existence: I am a marijuana addict and cannot, under any circumstances, allow THC to enter my bloodstream. Every moment of every day, consciously or unconsciously I choose not to get high, not to layer my awareness with a drug, not to step out of recovery and into addiction. I make this decision, in my morning meditation, when I brush my teeth, when I sit down with coffee after porridge and fruit. I make this decision, when I start my car, back out of the driveway, and head off to work. Every time I refuse to allow my diseased thinking patterns to rule my actions, I choose life over death. Daily meditation helps me to do this; it helps me to develop the ability to be alert and let go of thoughts that could lead me to relapse.

Final thought: Daily meditation trains my mind to notice and nurture thoughts that deepen my recovery.

My mantra is:

"Do not push away.

Have an open mind, an open heart;

Be open to everything;

Be awake and alert; not sleeping or dozing.

Be alive; not dead."

June 22

Spiritual Awakening

"By the grace of a Higher Power, we are given the gift of recovery. For most of us, recovery is a process that goes from awareness to awakening. We have many spiritual experiences before we have the permanence of a spiritual awakening as a result of growth from these Steps."

- Life With Hope, second edition, page 63

The gift of recovery occurs only when I keep coming back and when I put in the work, no matter how many times I may succumb to yet another relapse. I've spent several years in these rooms, gaining some clean time here and there, but never fully committing to the program, nor finishing the Twelve Steps, nor receiving a spiritual awakening, until now. As I have stayed clean for the longest time yet, I now know what this program can do. I was relentless enough to keep coming back, attempting to put my life back together after the last bottom that I hit. Three years later, I am still clean.

I had a spiritual awakening as the result of these Steps. I knew the miracles that could happen if I kept working the program. My greatest miracle was that I was living in a house full of stoners for the first nine months of my recovery. Most days, I would find weed on the floor and my roommate's bong on the table, coupled with a lighter. I had the ability, through my Higher Power giving me strength, to resist the temptations. I made it through practically the first year with temptation staring right at my face. There was no other way I could have done this on my own. My Higher Power gave me the tools I needed to stay clean in an addict's worst nightmare. It is through these Steps and the guidance of God that I was able to remove my obsession of using.

Final thought: Today, I will keep coming back, because it works if I work it.

June 23

The Fallacy of "Lightweight"

"It is very difficult to go to a meeting and be called a 'lightweight' by the other addicts when you are absolutely despondent about what is happening to your life and are trying frantically to get clean."

- Why Marijuana Anonymous, MA pamphlet

It is indeed very tragic that this belief that marijuana is non-addictive still permeates our society. Anyone who has the disease of addiction has earned a seat in these rooms. Marijuana addiction is often a death of a thousand cuts; it chips away at me until I find myself spiritually bankrupt. Spiritual bankruptcy is common across all addictions. One is no more or less "real."

Early in sobriety, before I knew MA existed, I would attend meetings of other fellowships and hear stories that frankly sounded nothing like mine. I identified with that "rock bottom" feeling, but I struggled to relate to the details of those stories. I personally was never made to feel unwelcome, but I couldn't shake the feeling that I was somehow different. I have heard stories of fellow marijuana addicts who were singled out in other meetings, one who was even told to leave. I deserve to feel welcome. The rooms of MA provide a space where I can openly share my stories without fear of ridicule and where I can relate to those around me.

Final thought: Today, I seek community that lifts me up. Today, I know that I am an addict.

June 24

Powerless

"We are powerless over marijuana in all its forms. Until we admitted our powerlessness, denial kept us from realizing how unmanageable our lives had become."

- Life With Hope, second edition, page 3

When I was new to MA I learned that I was powerless over marijuana and all mind-altering drugs including alcohol. I came to understand that once the substance entered my body, I wanted more of it. I could not control it. This had been my experience before coming to the program, so it was easy to comprehend. Over the years, I have realized that I am powerless over things outside of myself as well. This includes my partner's actions, traffic, and what my co-worker chooses to do.

When I forget that I am powerless over these things, my life becomes unmanageable because I will become overly frustrated and attempt to exert my will to change things. This is when I need to talk with my sponsor or a fellow in the program to be reminded about what actions I can take that will be helpful rather than hurtful. One example of an action that I implement is to surrender to my Higher Power. When I remember that I am powerless over these things I relax, because there isn't anything for me to do except turn it over to my Higher Power and that brings me a lot of serenity.

Final thought: Today, when I feel agitated by someone or something I will remember that I am powerless over it and then let it go.

June 25

Facing My Feelings

"Do you use marijuana to avoid dealing with your problems or to cope with your feelings?"

- The 12 Questions of Marijuana Anonymous, *For The Newcomer*, MA pamphlet

Feelings have always been difficult for me. I grew up an emotional child, in a household where feelings were unacceptable, so I learned to suppress my feelings on the outside. I grew a constant poker face and a monotone voice. You couldn't tell what I was thinking or feeling anymore. Inside though, I remained that emotional, anxious, and angry little kid.

Eventually I found marijuana, and it felt like the magical fix. I could laugh at things, let worry and anger disappear, and look at the world with wonder. I was creative and relaxed. I couldn't believe I waited so long to become a pothead. Flash forward eleven years and the magic was gone; pot was a tool of avoidance. I always had a feeling, thought, or emotion I couldn't face. If I was sad, anxious, or angry, I smoked; eventually I was smoking from the minute I woke up to the minute I fell asleep. This left me numb, vacant, and emotionally unavailable to so many precious moments for which I should have been present. Life was literally passing me by.

With recovery, I have the self-respect and dignity to face my feelings. I meditate, and pray to my Higher Power daily. I call fellows. I read the MA literature regularly. I attend several MA meetings a week, and have taken service commitments. I'm doing the Steps and I'm staying clean and sober, one day at a time. I could not have done this on my own. I needed this fellowship. I needed voices of shared experience, hands to reach out to, and ears to listen. I needed a group of loving marijuana addicts to remind me that I'm going to be OK, no matter what feelings are brewing inside.

Final thought: Today, I've found there are better ways.

June 26

Miracle of Recovery

"We asked our Higher Power for the willingness, strength and courage to look at ourselves honestly, fearlessly, and thoroughly."

- *Life With Hope*, first edition, page 18

Before marijuana took over, I had a dream to be a decent parent instead of "checking on something" in the basement, in the car, or in a walk around the block with a one-hitter. It's not easy to realize many of my dreams went up in smoke. I settled for the grandiosity of imagination. Subsequently, my goals were not met; life slipped away and it hurt to watch peers move ahead. For so many years in my life I was filled with pain and misery because I'd settled for drugs and behaviors I felt were wrong for me. I settled for activities that I thought I should do to please other people. I have been selfish and self-centered and accepted the pain that often results when I get my way. I've blamed other people for my troubles instead of looking for my part.

With recovery, I settle less now for pain and misery, though at times I feel it. Now, I try more to truly do what I feel is God's will for me. One way of looking at recovery is quitting that which causes me pain, like drugs and addictive behaviors, and doing what causes me to feel good about myself, like participating in 12-Step meetings, being loving, and being of service in spiritually fulfilling ways. I wish each and every one of us love and sobriety and the joy of living in fulfilling ways.

Final thought: Today, I can face the consequences of my "wasted" past, and move forward into a new day of recovery with sober choices. I can get myself back on track, and allow the miracle of recovery to gradually change my life for the better.

June 27

Came to Believe

"When we came to meetings and listened to others, we identified with the insanity of addiction as described by the members of the fellowship."

- *Life with Hope*, first edition, page 5

The ideology of insanity baffled me. I also believe that Higher Power is not separate or outside of me. In my workbook, I can cognitively reframe the Second Step so it is less religious sounding. Sanity means "of sound mind." For me, the power of connection with other cannabis addicts is a Higher Power.

As I listen to other addicts talk about what they did to use cannabis and the lengths they went through to continue to use cannabis, I am able to better understand how insane my behavior was in active cannabis addiction. Insanity is active addiction, which is the opposite of sound mind. When I used cannabis, my behavior was insane. In active addiction, my behavior was not in alignment with my intentions, values and morals of my authentic self.

In recovery, "we came to believe" that a power greater than our addiction could restore us to sanity. This greater power lives inside of me and within us all as a group of cannabis addicts. It starts within the mustard seed of faith "came to believe." Sound mind comes from the "came to believe" faith. This faith leads to an active, powerful daily decision to not use cannabis. I am restored in these 24 hours to sanity which is grounded in sound clean recovery. This affords me the experience and the opportunity to live in alignment with my authentic intentions and values.

Final thought: I choose to make a decision each and every day to continuously reprieve myself from active addiction; to not use cannabis, no matter what. Using is no longer an issue or an option.

June 28

We Recover

"We are all unique examples of how this program works, each of us with our distinct gifts to share. We take these steps for ourselves, not by ourselves. Others have gone before; others will follow. We recover."

- Life With Hope, first edition, page 69

There is no one way to work the program. There is no perfect recovery, no gleaming example of how to be the best fellow on earth. All one must do to be a part of our program is to not use, come to meetings, and take the Steps in one's own open, honest, and willing way. These are the lights that shine in our meetings; the ones that are just doing their absolute best with exactly what they have. Some days, that means crying through an entire speaker's share. Sometimes that means hitting a milestone with a grin. Sometimes that means being angry at our HP for being an addict in the first place. Sometimes, it's just showing up to the room in person or on Zoom, and melting in every word spoken, sitting in gratitude. We were unique in our addiction, and unique in the ways we experience our program, and every single day we get to recover just as we are, together.

Final thought: Today, I remember that the way I work the program is the way I'm meant to. One day at a time, one tear at a time, one mistake and inventory at a time. Today, I remember that I recover. Always.

June 29

Fears and Spiritual Growth

"Our awakening has come about as a result of a spiritual house cleaning, being aware of who we are, and cultivating a growing relationship with our Higher Power. That relationship can lessen the role of fear as the main source of motivation in our lives. We know that our needs will be met—perhaps not in the ways that we had hoped for, but in ways from which we can truly grow."

- Life with Hope, first edition, page 68

Sometimes, all I have to do to feel fear is look at my bank account. It seems that whatever number is in there, my fear-filled mind can label it "not enough" and then start spinning stories about looming poverty and a life on the streets. I think I deserve it all because of what a terrible person I am. What this program, and especially working the Steps, has given me is the ability to pause, and to observe my thinking. Working Steps Four and Five helped me to recognize those "patterns of thinking and behaving that can lead back to marijuana use." For if I get lost in that fear and those stories about my low self-worth, I will slip into despair. The pain and hopelessness will become so great that I will seek to self-medicate. No matter how long I stay clean, I am always capable of this, because my disease doesn't quit.

The key for me today is to maintain my spiritual condition, so that when those thoughts and fears arise, I can recognize them from my inventory. This gives me a little space to realize those thoughts are just projections of my fearful ego. What I can do is accept these thoughts and fears for what they are, perhaps as reminders of where I still have spiritual house-cleaning to do, and then work the Steps again. In this way, my fears can actually be opportunities for spiritual growth.

Final thought: Today, I will remember that my thoughts and fears are just projections of my ego, which will pass on like clouds. They don't separate me from the sunshine of the spirit unless I focus on them. Today, I will ask my Higher Power how these fears can help me grow spiritually.

June 30

Attitude Adjustments

"Our attitude has turned from denial, defiance, and belligerence to gratitude, humility, and a sincere effort to be of service."

- Life With Hope, second edition, page 48

When using pot every day, I could not fathom ever feeling grateful for anything. Life was hard, and all I could think about every day was how I was going to get more pot to stay stoned. For me, addiction was a negative outlook on life, focused on what I didn't have, and never giving thanks for what I did have.

When I came to recovery and I immediately lost the desire to use drugs and alcohol, I was amazed. The compulsion and obsession left me. I found meetings about gratitude to be annoying. I didn't understand when people said they were a grateful marijuana addict. What!? Then at five years clean, I experienced a very traumatic event which turned my life upside down. I never thought of using, but it took me several years to reestablish a connection with a Higher Power I didn't understand.

While grieving the changes that had occurred, I was able to focus on what was good in my life, and gratitude became my daily spiritual practice. Addiction is being negative, and recovery is about focusing on the good in my life. What I focus on grows, and today I know I am a very grateful marijuana addict. I am grateful for my sobriety and recovery, and for the 12 Steps that have changed my life in every way. My attitude has definitely changed from negativity to being able to focus on the positive.

Final thought: Today, I am grateful for my sobriety and my recovery, and all the blessings in my life. Gratitude is one of the most important tools in my recovery toolbox.

July 1

Self-Centeredness and Real Growth

"Working daily on our relationship with God, we discovered that our timetable for having our defects of character removed was not the same as God's timetable...We take action and leave the results of our request to our Higher Power."

- Life with Hope, first edition, page 34

Not just during my using career, but my entire life before, was based on self-centeredness. For years, I had been beating myself up over my moments of anger, hatred, impatience, and arrogance. During periods of using, but also while not using, I had only moderate relief from these ugly things. When I reached Step Seven I realized all of these things stemmed from self-centeredness. When I was angry it was because things didn't go the way that I wished they would have. When I was impatient it was because things weren't running on my timeline. When I was arrogant it was because I thought I was somehow better than the other person. I hated when people or things weren't the way I thought they should be. Me, me, me; it was all about me. All this time I had been looking at the symptoms of anger and impatience, but finally, thanks to Steps Six and Seven I see the real disease is self-centeredness.

With this knowledge, it's easier for me to treat my self-centeredness rather than trying to do whack-a-mole with all my defects. Through "progress, not perfection," I can accept my humanness, but I also recognize those moments when I'm being self-centered and at least attempt to correct myself. I can also take actions that are the opposite of self-centered: unselfish, humble, charitable, generous, and self-giving. Knowing that self-centeredness is my real problem, I can actually work on becoming that better, humble person whom I've always wanted to be.

Final thought: God, continue to take away my defects and help me take actions to continue to become a person who does Your will and not my own.

July 2

Challenging Stagnation in Recovery

"As we are so often told, recovery is not an event; it is a process."

- *Life With Hope*, third edition, page 31

When I feel I'm becoming a stagnant stoner in recovery, it may be the quiet voice of my Higher Power telling me that it's time to explore new opportunities for growth. Volunteering to take on a service position, reaching out to a newcomer I've not spoken to before, and going to different meetings are some of the ways I can begin to regenerate the desire to move forward in my program. This feeling of discontent can be transformed today, just as it has in the past, if I allow myself to see the multitude of opportunities before me.

Final thought: Today, I will breathe life back into my recovery by challenging myself to grow.

July 3

Running Out of Options

"We were then left with two alternatives: to stay as we were and continue using marijuana until we died, or to seek spiritual help."

- Life with Hope, first edition, page 5

When marijuana stopped being a part of my life, it felt empty and disorienting. I came to Marijuana Anonymous because I had to replace my everyday using with everyday recovery. I found that coming to meetings gave me a meaning and a purpose. I thought I had already tried everything and MA was my only hope. I heard the talk of a Higher Power and it scared me. I did not want to try this and fail because it was my last resource for sobriety.

Spirituality did not come at once, but when I started accepting help, coming to meetings, and applying the simple suggestions of this program, I realized I obtained what I've always been looking for: a new fulfilling way of life. It all started with being open to the idea of seeking help for sobriety since I cannot keep it on my own.

Final thought: Today, I have a simple choice to make between choosing freedom and sanity, or insanity by trying to go back to my old ways and expecting a different result.

July 4

Life-Long Process

"Addiction is a terminal disease that does not go into remission simply because we're not using. Constant vigilance is critical if we are to keep this disease at bay."

- Life With Hope, third edition, page 61

One of the most powerful pieces of wisdom I have heard at a meeting is "the good news is the monkey is off my back, the bad news is the circus is still in town." This is such an important analogy about the continuing need for me to maintain a strong recovery program. Even though I have been clean for a while, I can clearly see addictive thinking and behavior periodically coming into play in my life.

When I attend meetings and hear others share about their struggles with addiction, I am reminded of the fact that I may be a recovering addict but also that this is a life-long process. It is quite clear to me that it will be necessary for me to go to meetings for the rest of my life.

I am so grateful for having a clean life, and have made many wonderful friendships through MA meetings, so the idea of continuing to attend meetings is not a chore but is a very important component of having a happy and balanced life.

Final thought: I am convinced that going to meetings, being of service, talking with newcomers and other MA members, and talking with my sponsor are all crucial pieces of my continuing recovery.

July 5

Letting Go of Self

"We learned that the more we could let go of our selfishness and try to carry out what we perceived as God's will, the more we started to experience serenity in our lives."

- Life with Hope, first edition, page 33

Selfishness ruled my life in my addiction; I was too afraid and too desperate for control to give substantial thought to others and how my actions affected them. When I hit my bottom, I knew I had to change, but I didn't know what to change or how. The fellowship of MA showed me that change was possible, and that I didn't have to be afraid of letting go of my old ideas. Being of service showed me that I could make a positive difference in other people's lives, and enjoy doing it.

Most importantly, practicing the Twelve Steps of Marijuana Anonymous daily gives me a relationship with a Higher Power that frees me from the fears that drive my selfish thoughts and actions. As long as I am open to my Higher Power's will for me, and am willing to carry it out, I can experience a serenity I wouldn't have been able to conceive of when I was using.

Final thought: Today, I will try to recognize where selfishness still runs my life, and ask my Higher Power to free me from it.

July 6

Recovering My Feelings

"We found that when we denied, blocked, or buried our feelings, we usually behaved compulsively. Compulsive behavior can lead us to other addictions. When we acknowledged and accepted our feelings, we behaved moderately"

- *Life With Hope*, second edition, page 35

When I finally stopped smoking marijuana, I no longer had a way to escape from my feelings. I would remember events from my childhood or teenage years, and stuff them away by smoking. It was a very powerful way to get a reprieve from the negativity that would flood my brain on a regular basis. With my brain instead flooded with THC for years, I could not feel who I was. This was deeply disturbing to me but I kept going anyway, believing ignorance was bliss. I had goals and aspirations of becoming a professional filmmaker from an early age. I couldn't seriously pursue that goal while using, because it held me back from making deep connections with people.

I stopped smoking to follow my passion because it was either my dream or the drug, and all of a sudden I could feel again. This was scary, and in the time I've been in recovery I've had to process many years of backlogged emotional trauma and experiences. However what I didn't know, was how rewarding it would be to come to better understand myself and how I got here. I have had time and space to participate in my growth as a person because of the program, the Steps, sponsors, and hearing shares. In recovery, I know that I am safe and my feelings are safe too. I can enjoy and participate in a wide spectrum of experiences and emotions that make my life interesting and dynamic.

Final thought: Today, I like myself and I accept my feelings. With my recovery I am grateful to know myself better, to understand my feelings more clearly, and to be more effective towards achieving my goals with my MA toolbelt.

July 7

Character Defects

"The bottom line was a lack of humility. We could not see that good character and spiritual values had to come *first*. We had it backwards. We have found that material satisfaction and self-centered gratification of our desires are not the purpose of living."

- Life with Hope, third edition, page 30

Before I began the Step work, I would have said I'm the least selfish person ever. I was generous and giving and I loved hard. After doing Steps One through Six with honesty and discussion, I realized that I needed to ask my Higher Power to help me remove my selfishness in Step Seven. My desire to feel loved mixed with my codependency and enabling issues masked by staying high was a dangerously selfish combination.

Final thought: Today, even with all the pain and guilt, I think I am one of the "lucky" ones. If it wasn't for my addiction, I would not have worked these Steps and may have gone through life without spiritual growth.

July 8

Humility Leads to Serenity

"Humility is a simple request and a letting go."

- *Life With Hope*, first edition, page 34

Before recovery, I didn't know how to ask for help. I thought I had to figure everything out by myself. When I got to the Seventh Step and was told I needed to ask my Higher Power to remove my defects of character, I was stumped. Could I trust my Higher Power to make the changes I felt I needed to make? Humility means I step back from my problems, and I learn to trust that my Higher Power has my back and wants the best for me.

My first sponsor said I would never get rid of these "survival skills that no longer work," but that I would recognize them sooner. This has been my experience. I haven't completely lost my impatience, but I do recognize it quicker, and am able to make amends quicker too. I've heard it said that "humility is not thinking less of yourself, but thinking of yourself less." Humility does not mean we are less than or greater than; we are "right size" with our Higher Power and with others.

Final thought: Today, I see that humility is the key to serenity.

July 9

Seventh Step

"To take Step Seven, we needed to get out of God's way."

- *Life with Hope*, second edition, page 31

When I entered recovery, I never felt good enough, and I was always trying to be better, so that I would be loveable. I didn't know that I was OK. It took a lot of Step work to come to realize that I am loveable just as I am, and I don't need to be different to be OK. No matter how long I've been in recovery, every time the Seventh Step is a topic in a meeting, I am surprised to realize that once again I've forgotten that my job is not to try to fix myself. It's my Higher Power's job to heal me. My job is to ask my Higher Power to remove from me everything that stands in the way of me being a channel of my Higher Power's love and grace. I can relax then and know that change will happen, though not always according to my time.

Final thought: Higher Power, help me remember to let go of my arrogant self-criticism and turn over to you my shortcomings.

July 10

Merging My Will with My Higher Power

"The Third Step does *not* say, 'We turned our will and our lives over to the care of God, *as we understood God.*' It says rather, 'We made a decision' to do so. We didn't turn it all over perfectly or all at once. *We* made a decision. What an accomplishment this was! We made a decision; it was not made for us by marijuana, our families, a probation officer, judge, therapist, or doctor. We made it ourselves."

- Life With Hope, second edition, page 12

On re-reading this today, I was struck by the irony that the Step in which I accepted the care of my Higher Power was one in which I made a decision. I applied my will towards my recovery. This illustrates well how recovery requires both things: the things that my Higher Power cannot do for me, such as decisions; and the alignment of my will with my understanding of how my Higher Power wishes me to live. If I choose to make this decision today, there is no risk. I can change my mind and not do so tomorrow.

As an addict like many others in MA, my disease was full of decisions that I was too scared to make, and ones I habitually or lazily put off. This decision can be my chance to break the habit of procrastination and fear. I boldly made decisions to do what it took to get loaded. Now, I can boldly step up for today and try this on; turn it over, breathe, be grateful for what I have, and for the people who love me.

Final thought: Today, I am grateful for growth, freedom, joy, and happiness in my recovery.

July 11

Emotional Awareness

"One of the joys of being clean is the return of the full range of human emotions. Early on, we often confused feelings with defects of character; as our emotions returned with a new force, they frightened or disoriented us. We had not yet learned what to do with them."

- Life with Hope, second edition, page 35

Before I had quit weed and committed to the MA Twelve Step program, I feared having to feel my emotions. A huge part of my using revolved around escapism into my privately defined world to avoid intense negative emotions. Now that I participate in life with the help of the Twelve Steps, I embrace the vast spectrum of emotions. Being able to get to the other side of a negative emotion equals growth. To get to the other side, I must go through the emotion and thoroughly feel it.

The beauty of depression and anxiety is that they may not last forever, and there is always a lesson to be learned about the self. Why is it that some situation or person instills fear or sadness within me? What am I trying to hide from? What character defect is causing these emotions? Through deep introspection and meditation, the light creeps in; I uncover facets of myself that have been clouded by marijuana smoke. The program shines the light and takes away the darkness as spirituality improves through the Twelve Step program; soon these low points become few and far between.

Final thought: Today, I embrace my present emotion, for without sadness, there is no happiness.

July 12

A Reaching Hand in the Darkness

"We strive for progress, not perfection."

- Life With Hope, first edition, page 33

In my active years, I was always afraid; afraid of not being worthy of love, afraid of what others thought of me, and scared of not even being worthy of being alive. In the program and the fellowship, I met love and compassion. I met people who understood me, and who loved me when I couldn't love myself. I opened up to my Higher Powers, and today I am so grateful for all the help I have gotten, and am still getting. When I let go, and do my daily program, and trust in the process and in love, then I feel loved and safe, and I know that I am exactly where I am supposed to be.

Final thought: Today, I will surrender to my Higher Powers.

July 13

Humility

"Step Seven: Humbly asked God to remove our shortcomings."

- *Life with Hope*, first edition, page 31

For me, developing humility takes a long time. Humility involves seeing myself exactly as God sees me. I had to become humble in MA and that meant that I had to become teachable. Humility means that I accept reality. When I was using marijuana, I was stuck in a privately defined world of my own grandeur. Now that I am clean, I have to remember to stay in a fit spiritual condition. Being humble is being real, and by being real, I join the human race. Humility allowed me to be part of a fellowship, and that was what I was looking for my entire life.

Final thought: Today, I am free because I am humble.

July 14

The Master Gardener

"We asked for freedom from anything that limited our recovery and inhibited our relationship with our Higher Power."

- Life With Hope, first edition, page 31

Every day, I ask for the removal of any aspect of my character that blocks me from the love, grace, and guidance of my Higher Power. It is the times when I'm asking with genuine humility that I feel a shift in my perspective and an opening in my heart. I know that if I humbly ask and humbly listen, my life will continue to transform and grow.

In our literature, there is a reference to a "Master Gardener" who helps us remove the weeds in order to create space for our gardens to grow. In active addiction, I got lost in the weeds that took over my garden, and became disconnected from what my garden was meant to become. In recovery, I recognize those weeds are my shortcomings. I have to identify those shortcomings and actively participate in weeding them out and letting them go. I do this by being willing to change and humbly asking for these self-defeating aspects to be removed.

My hope is that through the transformational process found in the 12 Steps and a commitment to this fellowship, I will be able to grow into the person I was designed to be. As a result, I can be of greater service to others and live a more joyful, meaningful, and peaceful garden of life!

Final thought: Today, I will humbly ask and willingly listen to the wisdom of my Higher Power with an open mind and hopeful heart, trusting there is a divine plan for me.

July 15

Higher Power Love

"We strive for progress, not perfection."

- *Life with Hope*, first edition, page 33

I had a father who expected perfection. I was constantly criticized when I made a mistake. He felt that his way to do things was the right way and the only way. I tried very hard to do things the way that he wanted me to; I felt that then he would love me. I grew up feeling like a failure. I lost my self-esteem and self-respect. I withdrew from social situations. To try to be perfect is a losing situation: no matter how hard I tried, I could never be perfect.

When I came into the rooms of MA and heard the expression, "progress, not perfection," I was so relieved. I didn't have to try to be perfect anymore. I learned that my self-perceptions were not based on fact, instead, they were based on fear. I have learned to have faith instead of fear. With faith and acceptance, I have learned that my Higher Power loves me just the way that I am, and I am so grateful.

Final thought: Every day, I thank my Higher Power for my recovery.

July 16

A New Reality

"We are transformed from suffering addicts seeking relief from the grip of our disease into people who are able to be 'happy, joyous, and free.'"

- *Life With Hope*, first edition, page 63

Upon entering Marijuana Anonymous I listened to others talk about the reality of their using: pain, loneliness and fear. As I grew in the fellowship, I soon heard stories of a very different kind—the reality of sobriety. It is a reality of freedom and happiness, of purpose and direction, and of serenity and peace with the creator, ourselves and others.

When I attend MA meetings, I am reminded of this reality, over and over. I see it in the eyes and hear it in the voices of those around me. As I live the Steps of the MA program I find direction and strength. The joy of Marijuana Anonymous is that this new reality is available to me. As I grow in the fellowship of MA, I see that I was always real. I had just been looking at the outside.

Final thought: Today, I will be grateful that miracles have become everyday reality.

July 17

Finding a Higher Power

"Marijuana Anonymous gives us no definition of a power greater than ourselves. We practice spiritual principles, not religion. We have no theological doctrines. What we do have is a realization that we had never been able to stay clean on our own. We needed a Higher Power to do that."

- Life with Hope, third edition, page 10

When I first entered recovery, I had little belief that a Higher Power could "restore me to sanity," as it says in Step Two. I thought I could achieve sobriety on my own until I found I couldn't put down the pot, no matter how much I wanted to. Growing up, my father told me that people who believed in God and prayer were "brainwashed," and this clouded my perception of prayer and a Higher Power.

As I got clean and started searching for my own version of spirituality, I realized that people all over the world pray; even those who are non-theist. I've found that by asking for help from my Higher Power and by praying for others, I get more in touch with my own love and compassion, which has helped me realize that I never need to feel alone. No matter what I'm going through, there are countless others feeling the same way, in that same moment, all over the world. The people I've met in recovery remind me of this, too. They have helped me get in touch with a power greater than myself: the healing power of love, friendship and connection. I was so desperately craving this while I sat alone, stoned, watching TV, or scrolling through social media.

When I think about the support addicts offer to each other in the rooms of Marijuana Anonymous, I'm reminded that there is a power greater than myself, and it comes in many forms. We're free to believe in whatever Higher Power is meaningful to us.

Final thought: Today, I believe a Higher Power has been slowly working to restore me to sanity; a life which is balanced and allows me to act from a place of integrity.

July 18

Spiritual Progress

"Each day, we renew our commitment to spiritual progress in order to stay one step ahead of the progressive disease of addiction. We practice perseverance."

- Life With Hope, third edition, page 47

In working Steps Eight and Nine, my spiritual awakening is happening. As promised, I am finding a new freedom and a new happiness. Letting go of my anger and resentment by admitting them to another person really kicked off this process for me. I began to understand that fear and anxiety were ruling forces in most of my actions and relationships. By asking God to remove these and a few other negative qualities, I began the process of living a life that aligned my actions with my values. In taking the Steps to identify the harms that I have done to others and myself and making amends for them, I began putting this into action at a higher level.

Clearing away this wreckage has made room for a Higher Power to enter my life and guide me to the next right action. Checking in with my Higher Power daily through prayer and meditation, evaluating my behavior with others and making apologies or amends as needed, keeps my house in order. This clear space makes room for my Higher Power to show me what it is that I need to see and do next. Without the clutter of resentments, guilt and shame, there is space for gratitude, creativity, and deeply loving relationships.

Final thought: Today, I will take personal inventory to further my recovery and grow in connection with myself, others, and especially my Higher Power.

July 19

Humility is Key to Happiness

"To be humble is to be genuinely accepting."

- Life with Hope, first edition, page 36

I came into the rooms of Marijuana Anonymous because I felt so hopeless about my life. I could no longer control my marijuana smoking and I knew that I needed help. I knew that I needed support; I could not do this alone. I had to get the courage to say that I was a marijuana addict. I stopped denying my marijuana problem and knew that I had to surrender completely. Addiction, like depression, is a disease and it was necessary for me to admit that I was powerless over my marijuana use.

I learned to have faith in my Higher Power and it is so freeing to turn my life over to my Higher Power. With humility, I have a constant relationship with my Higher Power and the ability to ask for help. Humility is my key to serenity and happiness.

Final thought: I am filled with gratitude for what I have gained in recovery.

July 20

Spiritual Growth

"We find that if we give top priority on spiritual growth, it is less likely that self-will and character defects will pull us down."

- Life With Hope, first edition, page 60

By working the Steps, I come to accept a Higher Power's will. I lose my fear of the unknown. I am set free. Life is a series of changes, both large and small. Although I may know and accept this fact intellectually, chances are that my initial emotional reaction to change is fear. For some reason, I assume that each and every change is going to hurt, causing me to be miserable. If I look back on the changes that have happened in my life, I will find that most of them have been for the best.

I was probably very frightened at the prospect of life without marijuana, yet it's the best thing that's ever happened to me. Perhaps I've lost a job that I thought I'd die without but, later on, I found greater challenge and personal fulfillment in a new career.

As I venture forth in my recovery, I'm likely to experience more changes. I will outgrow old situations and become ready for new ones. With all sorts of changes taking place, it's only natural to grab hold of something familiar, and try to hold on. Solace can be found in a power greater than myself. The more I allow changes to happen at the direction of my Higher Power, the more I will trust that the changes are for the best. Faith will replace fear, and I will know in my heart that all will be well.

Final thought: When I am afraid of a change in my life, I will take comfort from knowing that God's will for me is good.

July 21

Acceptance

"In MA we at last found the courage to face the truth."

- *Life with Hope*, first edition, page 3

Accepting I have a problem with marijuana has been a challenge for me. My addiction is a "slow burn." I won't find myself being revived from an overdose; however, I found myself isolated and not managing my life after years of usage.

Accepting I am powerless over my addiction is part of the first step toward freedom. It also leads me to an acceptance of myself; the good, the bad, and the ugly. Acceptance may be difficult; however, in the fellowship of MA, I find others who relate to my stories and who share stories I can relate to. You are not alone! Fellowship with others who struggle with addiction to marijuana provides us support and encouragement. We, as a fellowship, accept one another. Even if I have trouble accepting myself, the fellowship accepts me until I can accept myself.

Final thought: Today, I am grateful for the acceptance shown by the fellowship of MA.

July 22

Power of the Deep Breath

"Some meditation methods suggest that we pay attention to our breath, as a way of quieting our mind."

- MA Workbook, first edition, 11th printing, page 53

For me, meditation is a time for reflection, to carve a few moments out of my day to intentionally slow down, practice presence, and to sit in conversation with the Highest version of myself. I also use meditation as an opportunity to receive what I refer to as "Divine Downloads."

Like many of us, I preferred to consume cannabis by smoking it (which I later realized was a form of deep breathing practice). I would fill my lungs as much as possible, holding my breath as long as I could. Then, with that exhale, all the cares of the world left me. So, when I quit smoking, I also quit intentional breathing.

As I came to Step Eleven, I found intentional breathing again by simply starting to focus on my breath and using it as an anchor, in preparation of, and during meditation. One day in meditation, I received one of these "Divine Downloads" and the message I heard was that I wasn't ever craving weed, I was craving a deep breath, and the sigh of relief that comes with it.

Final thought: As I breathe in "I let God" take care of my life, and as I breathe out "I let go."

July 23

Check Yourself

"Whenever we are suffering, we pause and check to see if we have been at fault."

- Life with Hope, first edition, page 36

Prior to coming into the rooms of Marijuana Anonymous, I looked to the world around me for the reasons that I experienced pain and suffering: my parents, my spouse, my siblings, my job...the list goes on forever. What I have learned in recovery is that in practically all of my life encounters where I experienced some sort of emotional pain, I have some part to play in my own suffering. This is very hard for me to come to grips with because I often saw myself as the one who had been wronged. This may be true. What is also true is that in any relationship where people are in conflict, there is almost always an opportunity for me to reflect upon "how I might have done something differently."

In recovery, I am fortunate to have a trusted advisor—my sponsor—with whom I can confide these types of issues, and discuss my suffering. Through working the Steps, and using specific events in my life as examples, I can see if I was an innocent victim or a willing collaborator in my suffering. If the latter is true, I am fortunate to have the tool of the amends process to alleviate my suffering and "amend" my behavior so the next time I encounter a similar situation I will be better prepared to act in a manner commensurate with my true nature.

Final thought: Today, I accept my part in my own suffering, and amend my behavior when necessary.

July 24

Action Steps

"After all, the faith we acquired by taking Step Three meant very little if we did not follow it with immediate action."

- Life With Hope, second edition, page 15

I am grateful that today my program is one of action and not talk, thoughts, or opinions. I've heard recovering people talk about some Steps being "action steps." One of the greatest gifts of recovery in my life is that it doesn't matter so much what I think as what I do. I have found that when I do the basic behaviors outlined in our program, I recover, one day at a time.

With the help and guidance of my sponsor and fellows, through whom my Higher Power communicates, I can seek and find the behaviors and actions that allow me to live the Twelve Steps on a daily basis. In this process, all Twelve Steps can become "action steps." Acts of service, acts of seeking connection with a Higher Power, acts of inventory, reading, fellowship, and meeting attendance, are all "action steps."

These simple actions are the keys which open the door to a life in which fear, self-centeredness, craving, and obsession might open the way, leaving me space to grow in my spiritual connection to myself, my fellows, my family, my communities, and my Higher Power.

Final thought: Today, let me have the willingness to act upon spiritual principles in all my affairs.

July 25

The Will of My Higher Power

"The basic ingredients of humility are unpretentiousness and a willingness to submit to a Higher Power's will."

- *Life with Hope*, first edition, page 31

One of the hardest concepts for me to get my arms around is "God's will for us." I trusted my best thinking and self-will, and it led me to addiction to marijuana and other substances. Now it is suggested that I submit to a Higher Power's will. The question that is often asked is, "How can I differentiate between my will and that of my Higher Power?" The answer is not easy, and the truth of my being is often found in the daily practice of prayer and meditation.

It has been said that prayer is speaking to my Higher Power, and meditation is listening to my Higher Power. Through this practice I am able to form a relationship with my Higher Power that yields peace, serenity, insight, and trust. I can start this practice at any time. There is no right way or wrong way to do this work. I can just be open, willing, and honest about my thoughts and feelings with my Higher Power, and say them out loud. I sit in the silence and listen and repeat daily.

Final thought: Today, I will speak my word to my Higher Power, and listen for the answer.

July 26

A Problem with Living

"We were not problem users whose problems went away when we threw away our stash. When we stopped using, we found we had a problem with living; we were addicts."

- *Life With Hope*, third edition, page 8

I have a living problem. This is both horrible and fantastic news; what is fantastic is that I'm not alone. I am not uniquely failing at the program because I sometimes still massively struggle with living life even though I have put the drugs down; not using doesn't cure all of my unhappiness.

I might wish it were true that once I put down the marijuana, my life instantly became spectacular and I began floating around on white robes, gravid with wisdom, and smiling at everyone. Instead, I found that I could be a real juvenile jerk at times, outright vicious, and self-pitying at others; only now I didn't have any drugs to blame!

I heard people in meetings say that their marijuana use had been a symptom of their disease and that their real problem was what was between their ears; that they suffered from uncontrolled bouts of thinking that stood to threaten their life at times.

Getting clean is a delicious miracle. I cannot do anything until I put the drug down. Once I do, though, I can't afford to stop and pat my own back for the next several decades or so. Getting clean gives me a fighting chance to change my life. I am an addict and that fact doesn't change when I turn away from marijuana.

Final thought: Today, I will remember that recovery is a delicious miracle that gives me a fighting chance to change my life.

July 27

A New Perspective

"The process of gaining this new outlook on life was a painful experience for most of us."

- Life with Hope, first edition, page 33

I have heard it said that the mind can be a very dangerous place. My thoughts can take me in a direction that is a challenge to my sobriety, and in many instances, take me back to old ways of doing and being which no longer serve me. Why is changing perspective so difficult for marijuana addicts like me? For one thing, when I have lived one way for so many years, it is hard to make a sudden radical change. Others have told me that they never had any positive influence to tell them there is another way to live. Ultimately, it really doesn't matter why. What really matters is how I can create positive change in my life.

Like the master musician, the elite athlete, and the expert craftsperson, as an addict I must practice recovery to gain a new perspective on life, and ultimately find a new way to live. My practice includes prayer, meditation, service, fellowship, and study. Our fellows can also teach us many other valuable practices that have helped them in their recovery like yoga, exercise, chanting, or drumming, and many other practices.

The practice of recovery leads to the building of useful life tools. The building of tools leads to new ways to live. New ways to live leads to new ways of thinking. New ways of thinking lead to an entirely new perspective.

Final thought: Today, I know, as I change my thinking, I change my life.

July 28

Peace and Gratitude

"By the time we have reached this Step, we are feeling peace and serenity, which replaced pain, fear, and desperation as the motivating forces in our lives."

- Life With Hope, first edition, page 59

When I was getting high, my idea of "peace" was to obliterate everything going on in my head. The problem was that I couldn't dull just the bad thoughts and feelings; I dulled everything. Inside, I was still tortured about my using and my unmanageable life. When I came to Marijuana Anonymous and got clean, with the support of the group and meetings, I found a new kind of peace. Once the obsession to use was lifted from me, I was free of the shame that went with my active addiction but all those thoughts and feelings came back. It was time to do the work of "spiritual housecleaning." When I did Steps Four and Five, I was able to realize I wasn't a horrible monster, just someone with a disease called addiction. This was a new kind of peace, self-acceptance.

Today, my idea of peace is being in that calm, quiet place in my center, knowing I am loved, whatever is going on outside. I can experience ups and downs, I can have positive and negative thoughts, and still be OK. This allows me to be present with what actually is going on, rather than off in a fog of thinking, or swept away by feelings. Especially when I work Step Eleven, it's precisely the moments of non-peace when I can stop, look within, and ask myself what's going on, what part of the spiritual house needs a little cleaning?

Final thought: Today, I will take some time to simply sit in peace and gratitude. I will be present with whatever is happening, inside and out. When thoughts or feelings arise, I won't seek to push them away, rather I will accept them as teachings.

July 29

A Power Greater Than Myself

"Once we admitted our powerlessness, we had to find a power greater than ourselves by which we could live."

- Life with Hope, second edition, page 5

I admit: my utter failure at life under the crushing obsession for marijuana.

I seek: a solution to freedom from my addiction.

I surrender: my incapable willfulness and confining judgments.

I accept: the guidance and success of those who preceded me.

I embrace: the journey toward a loving presence in my life.

I live humbly now by the principles of the Steps in service of the Greater Power.

Final thought: Today, I put principles into action.

July 30

No Excuses

"We become true partners with our friends and loved ones. With the help of a Higher Power, we respond positively to adversity."

- *Life With Hope*, first edition, pages 68-69

I hadn't come home for my first two Christmases in recovery. By the third year, I felt I was ready. I had better boundaries and a more solid connection to my fellows, sponsor, the Steps, and my Higher Power. The first thing I noticed is that I had changed, but my controlling family had not. Within mere days, I could feel myself being pulled back down into the molasses of their negativity, where my mom's growing rage awakened my own. One day, my mom got to me so badly with her constant criticism of me and her growing violence towards my dad (who's now wheelchair-bound), that I could feel myself wanting to do something drastic to make her stop. I couldn't believe how close I'd come to throwing away not only my recovery, but all my life's dreams, too.

I looked at my phone through tears, and a message was waiting for me from a fellow. We talked, which calmed down my pounding heart. In my notebook, I spotted words from my sponsor, "Don't try to out-crazy crazy." My first responsibility was to stay safe, serene, and clean. I took a full four days away from my family, regained my sense of self I'd been building in recovery, and returned stronger for when the next meltdown came (and oh, how it came). I was so grateful I hadn't thrown it all away, and let other people's bad behavior become my excuse to pick up.

Final thought: It feels good to develop level-headedness and discernment by being clean and, as the family scapegoat, to realize that perhaps all these years, I wasn't the crazy one!

July 31

Faith and Acceptance

"By starting to trust our Higher Power, we cleared the way for growth and recovery. Now we no longer have to rely on the weak force of self-will to solve our problems. Faith and acceptance are our new solutions."

- Life with Hope, first edition, page 13

Having faith requires believing in something without having proof that it exists. In recovery, it is necessary to believe in something greater than myself. It is difficult to relinquish control, but it can be exhausting to swim against the current. The current is a force greater than myself, and I am too weak to fight against the tide, so I learn to surrender.

To let go, and have the tide take over, is the only way to let the force of what is greater than me, my Higher Power, work. I am focused on one tiny grain of sand, but God, as I understand God, has a view of the entire beach. I may not understand now, but I trust that God knows what is best for me, for my growth and for my recovery.

Final thought: Today, I will have faith, and accept that my will and desires are limited to the view of one tiny grain of sand, and my Higher Power sees the whole beach.

August 1

Amends to Myself

"Step Eight was the beginning of the end of our isolation."

- Life With Hope, second edition, page 42

Before recovery, self-care was a foreign concept. I worked the Steps with my sponsor, and when I got to Step Eight, I was told to put myself at the top of my amends list. Upon reflection, I could see how much I had harmed myself in my addiction. I cut myself off from my dreams, my ambitions, my connections with others, and especially my connection with myself.

I make amends to myself by taking good care of my body, my emotions, my spiritual health, and my recovery. I know that I must keep my recovery a priority in my life. If I'm not clean, I will lose all the blessings that have come to me since I gave up marijuana, and surrendered to my powerlessness over marijuana. I can never forget I'm an addict, and I need meetings, a sponsor, working the Steps, and a community of fellow addicts to have a peaceful, joyful, and serene life. I make amends to myself every day by staying close to the program, and close to my friends in recovery. I also stay close to my Higher Power, which keeps me "right" inside.

Final thought: I make amends to myself through living a life of recovery, one day at a time.

August 2

Meditation

"Prayer and meditation are a real source of power and strength in living our program."

- *Life With Hope*, first edition, page 56

Mindfulness practice is the basis for my meditation. When I remain in the present moment and as conscious as I can be of what's happening within me and around me, then I can trust in the presence of a power greater than myself.

When I was in active addiction I was living a double life. On the outside I was trying to show the world that everything was OK. Yet on the inside, there was this person screaming about the insanity of my life and no one could hear me. I wanted to stop the cycle of my marijuana use; yet again, every day I needed to smoke marijuana to try and deal with my life. Marijuana had stopped working years ago but I kept using, thinking it would stop that deafening silence, but the scream in my head kept me up at night and kept telling me I was no good; telling me I was no good, that I wasn't worth it.

In recovery, I have learned that the silent scream can be silenced by sharing at meetings, sharing with my sponsor and working the program of recovery.

Final thought: Today, I will remember the importance of sharing with my sponsor and working the program of recovery.

August 3

It Works If You Work It

"We say, 'we take' these Steps, not 'we took' them, because we live these Steps continually."

- *Working the Program*, MA pamphlet

The only requirement for membership in our program of Marijuana Anonymous is a desire to stop using. In my case, the only requirement for getting clean and staying clean is a willingness to do the work this program requires of me.

It is not enough for me to have worked the Steps, I must continue to work the Steps. It is not enough for me to do service work, I must continue to do service work. It is not enough for me to reach out to the newcomer, or even someone who has been in the program longer than I have—I must continue to do these things.

It is not enough for me to know marijuana is bad for me, not enough for me to not want to use anymore, to be done with it, or to despise my using with every fiber of my being. I am an addict, and I must be reminded, daily, that I am incapable of stopping without the help of a Higher Power and the fellowship of addicts like me.

"This program is not easy, but it is simple." Anything that is not easy requires hard work. While there are many, many ways of working a program, once I find a program that works for me, I must work at it hard to obtain my daily reprieve.

Final thought: Today, I will do the work needed for me to stay clean.

August 4

Isolation

"Isolation and sulking are simply subtle ways to be prideful and vengeful. We gain the ability to think before we act."

- *Life With Hope*, second edition, page 50

The promises of the Twelve Steps come true for me, sometimes quickly, sometimes slowly. I need to work at them, and they don't all come overnight. With good, orderly direction (GOD) to guide me, I slowly incorporate spiritual principles into my life. These spiritual principles, such as honesty, open-mindedness, and willingness, the HOW of the program, help me become something better.

Before recovery, I isolated, even when around people, and I always spoke whatever was on my mind, never thinking first. By working the Twelve Steps, the promises have come true for me, albeit quite slowly. Ironically, by focusing on myself and growing, I can become more focused on helping others.

Final thought: Today, I can have fewer resentments towards others, and more reasons to appreciate myself.

August 5

Going to Extremes

"We need counsel because, as addicts, we so often go to extremes."

- Life With Hope, first edition, page 40

Now that I have some time living "one day at a time," I sometimes get a little surprised when I find myself going to extremes. I am fully aware that "none of us are saints" but the intensity of my "great ideas" can really get going some days. I stay close to my program pals and run some thoughts past them. I try not to be defensive and really listen to those who have my best interests and I trust to be truthful.

A pattern for me is when I get overwhelmed, I sometimes add on more "great ideas." I have days when I totally forget to "let go and let God" and "keep it simple." When I feel that I have to "fix everything and everyone," I know that my "EGO" is ramping up because I'm "Edging God Out." I stop, breathe, pray, and try to remember what serenity feels like. I find gratitude and not try to tackle all my problems at once.

Eventually, I can bring myself back into balance with some humor and God's help. I have been given this wonderful miracle of being clean and I can accept the rest of reality with a hopeful heart.

Final thought: Today, I know I can "start my day over" at any given moment.

August 6

Relinquishing the Illusion of Control

*"Higher Power, I have tried to control the uncontrollable for far too long.
I ask that you take this burden from me."*

- *Life With Hope*, second edition, page 13

One of the symptoms of my disease of addiction is that I feel the need to control everything. For years I controlled how I felt by numbing myself with marijuana. As I've heard it said in meetings, once I'm clean I'll get to feel everything. I absolutely need the Steps to clean house, learn how to feel my feelings, and trust my Higher Power.

I've struggled on and off with faith in a Higher Power. Recently I read that faith is like everything else, it appears to come and go. My faith never really leaves me. I remember hearing early on that if I don't feel connected to my Higher Power, it's me who's moved. In actuality, I cannot be separate from my Higher Power.

Just like my disease is never gone from me, my desire to control also has never left. Sometimes it sits in the corner trying to figure out what I need to do to fix a person or a situation, when really what I need to do is turn to my Higher Power and ask for help. It helps to remember that control is an illusion. I don't really have control; I just think I do.

I also need to ask for help from my sponsor, friends in recovery, and by going to a meeting. Those are the ways I get reminded that my Higher Power cares for me and wants me to be happy, joyous, and free. I can then remember that it's safe to turn over my will and my life, and that I do not have to control everything to be OK.

Final thought: Today, I remember that I can relinquish control to a loving, caring Higher Power.

August 7

When I Use, My Life Is An Eraser

"We therefore open our doors to any addict who has the simple desire to stop using marijuana, hoping that they can find what we have found in MA."

- Life with Hope, second edition, page 78

As I fell asleep last night, I reflected on the insanity of my using. How tragic that I spent years stoned, unaware that I could not stop or how I was ceasing to live my life. Day after day, I used pot to numb myself every waking moment, then grace entered. It had been knocking on the door for several years, telling me I needed to quit. How often I would say "this is my last bag" only to get another.

Finally, I must have shared my desperation with someone who referred me to a meeting. I had been trying to stop on my own, and now I could see people, other addicts like me, supporting each other, doing recovery together. The shackles of addiction fell off me, and I have never felt the compulsion to use again. I know that I have a life today because I'm present for it, and not numbing myself. I know that if I were to use again, I might not get another chance at recovery, and the life that I love would be erased. I know that recovery, and my life, is lived one day at a time, and I am grateful to be present for each day.

Final thought: Today, I am grateful for the grace that keeps me in recovery, doing what others do to stay clean.

August 8

Six Months Clean

"Do not be discouraged, none of us are saints. Our program is not easy, but it is simple. We strive for progress, not perfection. Our experiences, before and after we entered recovery, teach us three important ideas: That we are marijuana addicts and cannot manage our own lives; That probably no human power can relieve our addiction; and That our Higher Power can and will, if sought."

- How It Works, *Life With Hope*, third edition, page 193

Today, I am six months clean of marijuana. I never thought I'd make it here. I am thankful for my recovery and appreciative of my own work, but I also acknowledge that it wouldn't be possible without this program and this fellowship. Six months clean; this seemed entirely unbelievable to me less than six months ago. The transformative power of Marijuana Anonymous, of the Twelve Steps, and of the fellowship are what made it possible. It makes the unbelievable possible; that's why I keep coming back.

Final thought: Today, recovery means being surrounded by people who love me, shelter, employment, and my sanity.

August 9

The Value of Outreach

"We reach out to other addicts. We approach and make ourselves accessible to newcomers before and after meetings and during breaks... When we are having a bad day, our self-absorption diminishes when we take the time to reach out."

- Life with Hope, second edition, pages 64-65

Being in these rooms, I've learned the value of outreach. This includes reaching out to others when I need support, reaching out to others when I believe they need support, or being available when others reach out to me.

Gratefully, I've come to a miraculous jumping off point in my recovery to pursue endeavors that I never dreamt were possible. Simultaneously, I have found an amazing way to still be of service and share my experience, strength, and hope. This is by making phone calls and sending texts to newcomers and old friends in the program who I know are struggling. The beauty of the fellowship is there are always fellows to lean on who are not necessarily our sponsor, but who can help carry us through. It is important for me to remember that without a title, I can still be a tremendous source of hope.

With sobriety, I've been paradoxically freed from that relentless craving which in turn frees me up to be available to others' needs, inside and outside of these rooms. I've learned to live less selfishly. Only by giving it away, do I get to keep my recovery.

Final thought: Today, I will take my eyes off myself and put them on other people.

August 10

A Message of Hope and Promise

"Our message is one of hope and promise that any addict can stop using marijuana, lose the obsession and desire to do so, and find a new way of life by following spiritual principles one day at a time."

- Life With Hope, first edition, page 82

Before coming to Marijuana Anonymous, every day was filled with despair and hopelessness. I tried many times to stop using marijuana and could not get through withdrawal symptoms. After praying to my Higher Power for months and witnessing a miracle in someone else's life, I was curious if my Higher Power could help me make it through withdrawal symptoms and bring me out of intense suffering.

I found Marijuana Anonymous online and reached out in pain and desperation. When I dialed into my first phone meeting, I heard other real people who had gotten through withdrawal and had various lengths of clean time. I heard their obsession had been lifted. Through prayer, the experience, strength, and hope I heard in the meetings, and contact with other marijuana addicts, I not only got through withdrawal, but came to believe I could be restored to sanity. I found a sponsor and started working the Steps.

My experience working the Marijuana Anonymous program has yielded more healing, serenity, and freedom than I could ever have imagined when I was stuck in the depths of using marijuana.

Final thought: Today, I share my message of hope, sobriety, freedom, and healing with others who seek recovery.

August 11

Surrender to Hope

"All we need is to maintain an open mind and a hopeful heart."

- Life with Hope, first edition, page 7

I was hurt for so long by my unidentified hopelessness. Everything was crushing and bigger than a positive thought. I was uncomfortable with the idea of "God restoring me to sanity." A Higher Power doing so was slightly less intimidating; but I was still unwilling to let go, unwilling to turn my will and my life over to this unknown entity. My sponsor said, "you don't have to say yes, just stop saying no;" that did it.

Once I stopped saying no, a Higher Power came into my life and heart, giving me a life beyond my wildest dreams. When I reached for help before I found Marijuana Anonymous, I was turned away and I stopped reaching. Older now, I confided my hopelessness to others. My Higher Power shows me how to get out of bed; how to try things that I don't know how to do.

Final thought: Today, I am able to surrender to hope, instead of hopelessness.

August 12

Honesty

"Our program is not easy, but it is simple."

- How It Works, *Life With Hope*, first edition, page 103

"Keep it simple," what does that mean? When I came into recovery my life was anything but simple. I had to feed my addiction around the clock. I took whatever measures were needed, regularly lying; I had to. The freedom that comes with recovery is beautiful! I didn't think it was possible and had absolutely no idea where to start.

I just needed a baby step to get me going. It started with honesty. I had to be honest with myself that living in the prison of addiction was no longer working for me. I had to be open to a solution and willing to try. I love the acronym HOW, Honesty, Openness, and Willingness; this is how I got sober. If I continue to be rigorously honest and do the next right thing, my life is free of shame and remorse. When I'm free of the "ick" feelings, life is beautifully simple!

Final thought: Today, I try to be honest, it's simple but not easy!

August 13

Carrying the Message

"We are now in a position to truly carry the message, in a powerful and joyful way, to fellow addicts who are still suffering. This is possible because we ourselves have become living proof that the program works."

- Life with Hope, second edition, pages 63-64

Once upon a time, there were addicts who couldn't stop smoking pot, though they didn't enjoy it anymore. The daily craving overrode their frustration. They couldn't imagine what life would be like without pot. They must've told someone of their plight, because they found a meeting and started to get a glimmer that there were others like them, who'd been addicted but now were free of this substance. The talk about God was abhorrent at first, but the prospect of being free was greater, so they continued to go to meetings, and slowly understood what the Steps could do, and that it was OK, even necessary, to let others help them on this journey. To be free of the constant craving was the first of many wonderful gifts.

Final thought: May I today remember the freedom I enjoy, and reach out my hand to the still-suffering addict.

August 14

Letting Go of Blame

"We spent a great deal of energy blaming others for our problems."

- *Life With Hope*, third edition, page 3

During the height of my marijuana addiction, I actively blamed others in my life for my problems, especially my family. "No one has as crazy a family as I do," I would tell people. Criticizing others for my troubles allowed me to justify my continued, daily using. I collected and savored resentments like the shake at the bottom of a bag of weed, not knowing how much both were making my life miserable. I relished the competitive nature of comparing my life with others. It fed my desire to want to "win" arguments and fights. I would encourage friends to share their family stories, then I would counter with an even worse one. "See how much worse my family is than yours!?" I wanted sympathy and empathy, but mostly I just wanted to feel vindicated. Deep down, I wished I had a normal family and I expected them to treat me better.

In Marijuana Anonymous, I learned that expectations were the seeds of resentment, and that other people's opinions of me were none of my business. What was my business was my opinion of others, and those needed to change. Working the Steps, I stopped finding fault in others and instead looked at what I brought to my relationships. All the energy I had expended focusing on how others had harmed me only hurt me in the end. Once I looked at all my resentments, and my role in them, only then was I able to let go of blaming others and clean my own side of the street.

Final thought: Today, I no longer find fault with what others say and do. Instead, I work on letting go of my character defects, turning to the fellowship and my Higher Power for guidance.

August 15

I Am An Addict

"Casual or social marijuana use is not addiction. Addiction manifests in a compulsion to seek and take the drug, loss of control over limiting intake of the drug, diminished recognition of significant problems, emergence of a negative emotional state, craving, chronicity and relapse...Once one crosses the line into addiction, the brain is altered in a dramatic fashion."

- A Doctor's Opinion about Marijuana Addiction, MA pamphlet

Relapse has been an important part of my story. It was hard for me to stay clean the first time I tried to stop because I saw my friends in college smoking pot without having the negative consequences that I experienced. I smoked again, thinking that with the knowledge I had gained during my time in the rooms, I would be able to better manage my use. Before long, the same problems quickly emerged with using compulsively, by myself, all day every day. The anxiety and depression quickly followed.

When I came back into the rooms it was important for me to recognize that I am not like my friends; I am an addict, and no amount of time in the rooms is going to change it. The *Doctor's Opinion* tells us about the changes that happen to our brain after sustained long periods of marijuana use. More convincingly, the fellow marijuana addicts I encounter at meetings testify about how they have been able to find a life that is better than they could have imagined before they were in recovery. Also, they tell me that life in recovery is more satisfying than life with marijuana.

Today, I am kept clean by a realization that I am fundamentally different than my friends who can use in a safe and controlled manner. The rewards I continue to reap every day as I seek to live life on a spiritual basis reinforce my recovery.

Final thought: Today, I will not use, no matter what, because there is nothing that is so bad that a joint won't make it worse.

August 16

Living in an Unrealistic Delusion

"Step One is about honesty, about giving up our delusions and coming to grips with reality."

- Life With Hope, second edition, page 1

Oh reality, what an uncomfortable foreign concept you were, I'll escape instead. Honesty with others? Sometimes; honesty with myself? Completely incapable; delusion, that was my reality. Before coming into MA and working the program, I didn't know left from right or up from down. I thought I did; I thought I knew everything, which was far from the truth.

Step One, was the beginning of the healing that I so desperately needed. It was the jaws of life that ungripped my slave-like addiction to marijuana. Now, I am able to face reality as honestly as I can while slowly replacing the delusional thoughts that still sometimes occupy space in my brain. I don't do it perfectly, but every day that I'm alive and sober I get to try. This results in a life that doesn't require escaping, a life worth living.

Final thought: Today, I will try my best to be honest while I live life in real time and not escape into my delusional thoughts.

August 17

Freedom from the Bondage of Self

"By starting to trust our Higher Power, we cleared the way for growth and recovery. Now we no longer have to rely on the weak force of self-will to solve our problems."

- Life with Hope, first edition, page 13

I've heard, "I'm an ego maniac with an inferiority complex." I can relate to this statement. I seem to be on both sides of a spectrum of self-esteem. At times, I think of myself as "holier than thou" or some great knowledgeable person who others look up to; at other times I think of myself as a worthless loser. I have learned through the program that my self-centered thinking is at the core of this dichotomy. In the past, I felt responsible for much of what was going on outside of me and developed a belief that I could control it.

In my years of recovery, I have learned that I am responsible for my actions and God is responsible for the results. I must focus on the right action for me and not let fear, or desire for results, affect that focus. I am trying to learn humility, to let go of my self-centered egotistical thinking, see others as fellow travelers on this spiritual path, and recognize God as the one in charge. My bad habit of judging people (including myself) has diminished as I work the program. I am slowly learning to accept myself, others, and life as they are, instead of expecting them to be something I have conceived.

Life continues to turn out so much different from my ideas and plans of how I wanted it to be and this is very painful at times. I am, however, experiencing levels of joy and fulfillment that I could never have dreamed of, and it is clear now that God knows what is best for me.

Final thought: Today, I like myself most of the time. I still experience periods of self-hatred and inflated ego, but they are less frequent now and the duration is shorter. MA is saving me from the bondage of self and I am grateful.

August 18

Forever Grateful

"We have grown free and joyful."

- *Life With Hope*, third edition, page 45

Living as an addict and living in recovery is as different as night and day. My life as an addict became a descending spiral that entrapped my body, mind, and spirit. Admitting my powerlessness over marijuana and accepting that my life had become unmanageable was essential to being set free of the trap of my addiction. I had been told that the First Step is the only Step that I need to work 100 percent of the time. I was also told that my recovery required that I become honest, open-minded, and willing to in order to reap the numerous benefits of the MA program. My Higher Power, the fellowship and the MA program have set me free. I now try to practice the principles of the program to grow along spiritual lines.

Final thought: I am grateful for the rewards received by practicing the principles of the MA program in my daily affairs.

August 19

Gratitude List

"We were full of fear. Those fears stopped us from doing what needed to be done. Some of us were delusional; we lived in a private world that no one else shared. Perhaps we considered suicide, were otherwise depressed, or found ourselves unable to interact with other people. Maybe we were desperately lonely. For many of us, our self-pity became anger at the world for mistreating us and, for some, this anger escalated into rage."

- Life with Hope, second edition, page 16

When I wake up each morning, I find negativity running freely throughout my mind. My old way of thinking and behavior would have me focusing on this negativity and starting a mindset cycle of self pity and "poor me, I'm a bad person, I'm not rich enough, people don't like me, I haven't achieved what I want in life," and on, and on.

When I work my recovery program I engage my gratitude list. There are so many things for me to be grateful for right now. I am clean this morning, I am alive. I can think. I have a place to sleep. I have a program where I have friends to listen to me and help me. I care enough about myself to be in recovery. The wildfire of hopelessness that had seemed overwhelmingly depressing soon becomes significantly diminished, quenched in a waterfall of gratitude.

The score of my life flips from an addict mindset to an enlightened attitude of strength and power. I am now easing into a beautiful day.

Final thought: Today, I will awake and think of what I am grateful for. The negative thoughts that used to plague me will not run my life.

August 20

A Handbook for Living

"It's as though I finally got that 'How To' manual I always wanted when I was younger."

- Lightweight, *Life With Hope*, second edition, pages 186-187

This quote is from the story Lightweight in *Life with Hope*. I'd never wondered about a how-to manual growing up, but I related to this idea all the same. I grew up thinking everyone knew more than me. When I had a dilemma before recovery, I would ask eight different people what I should do, and get eight different answers. Only after working the Steps, did I begin to trust that I have my own answers, instead of relying on someone else.

I came to recovery unable to trust anyone or anything; mostly I couldn't trust myself. I'd wanted to quit marijuana years before I was able, and I was constantly making other people my Higher Power. Eventually, working the program, and forming real friendships with other recovering addicts who were safe, has helped me learn how to trust myself. I finally got the tools I didn't know I needed to help me learn to live a happy, joyous, and free life, clean, one day at a time.

Final thought: Today, I have a program and a fellowship to help me live life on life's terms.

August 21

11th Step Meditation

"Prayer and meditation are a real source of power and strength in living our program."

- Life with Hope, first edition, page 56

One day, I was on my knees picking out bits of pot that had fallen onto an upholstered chair seat. I realized, with some shame, that marijuana was the only thing that would get me on my knees—and had become my Higher Power. Shortly after coming into recovery, a spiritual advisor insisted that I meditate on a regular basis, which is probably the most helpful advice I have ever received. I have learned that when I am faithful to an Eleventh Step discipline of meditation, my life is different. I find that I have more serenity; that I am able to relate more healthily to the people around me, to the circumstances of my life, and to the world.

Today, I still can't define my Higher Power with anything more specific than "love" and "strength." I find it's all I need. The more connected I am to my Higher Power, the more connected I feel to other people and to creation. I don't know how or why it works—but it does.

Final thought: Today, I will spend some time in meditation. I will rest in my Higher Power.

August 22

See it. Say it. Do it. Be it.

"We recover."

- *Life With Hope*, first edition, page 69

The length of time in recovery is less important than the quality of recovery. Taking healthy risks, pushing boundaries, getting out of my comfort zone, expanding my skills; this is how I am recovering a life I wanted. I had to see others model things. I'd say "I want to do that," or "can I do that?" I would do it, and see how it felt. Thank you Higher Power, for giving me the power to take the next right step.

Final thought: Today, I can embrace growing new parts of my potential.

August 23

An Open Mind

"It is not necessary to acquire a major God Consciousness to be able to cease using. All we need is to maintain an open mind and a hopeful heart."

- Life with Hope, second edition, page 7

Having entered MA as an atheist, I have a long history of resisting the Step Two challenge of coming to believe in a Higher Power. Even after hundreds of meetings and two years of being clean, skepticism remains one of my core values. I approach Step Two not by abandoning skepticism, but by suspending it from time to time, to see if doing so improves my life. It often does. Although I don't believe that anyone listens to my prayers, I find great power in the act of prayer itself. I sometimes think of it as playing a trick on my ego—tricking it into getting out of the way for a while, so I can deal with whatever problem to which it might be contributing.

Though I started out thinking of my Higher Power as simply the other people in MA, I now see it more broadly as the state of consciousness fueled by my connections to those people. This allows me to carry my Higher Power out of the meetings and into the rest of my life. I feel its presence when I do a good job at work, call my parents to catch up with them, or help a stranger on the street who asks for directions. It's the state of consciousness in which I do the right thing, and channel serenity into my life.

Final thought: Through this approach to Step Two, I stay true to my values without letting rigidity hinder my recovery. Marijuana broke me; in light of that, I'm okay with bending a little on the spiritual stuff.

August 24

The Beauty of Recovery

"Recovery does not happen all at once. It is a process, not an event."

- Life With Hope, third edition, page 5

Recovery is beautiful and painful. Becoming the best version of myself is amazing and messy. There are aspects of my life that have improved so much and there are some things that have kind of fallen apart. I know with practice and patience, everything will fall into place; however, before it can fully get better it must also fall apart. I'm not the person I thought I would be and that gets frustrating. I want it to come quickly, but that is not how recovery works.

At this point, I must accept my limitations. I must accept that I am only human and that it took many years for my life to unravel, so it is not probable that I can put it back together in only a couple of months. Things will come in time. My energy will slowly replenish. My spirituality will heal if I practice it. My relationships will improve as I do, and my life will flow as it's meant to. Any day that I am clean is a blessed day.

I trust that the plan for me may look differently than the one I had for myself and with direction my recovery is ever blossoming. I put my faith in my Higher Power.

Final thought: Today, I ask to be granted the patience and understanding to know that I am exactly where and who my Higher Powers wants me to be.

237

August 25

Primary Purpose

"Our primary purpose is to stay free of marijuana and to help the marijuana addict who still suffers achieve the same freedom."

- MA Preamble, *Life with Hope*, first edition, page *xi*

Before I started down the path of recovery, the idea that I would discover a "primary purpose" for my life always seemed like a fantasy. I had to stop smoking weed, and I couldn't even do that. I was hopeless.

It was only after I entered recovery, admitted my powerlessness over marijuana and other mood and mind-altering substances that I began to discover who I was. It took all the struggles and pain my life could serve up before I really admitted I had no idea how to live life, how to stop smoking, or how to live up to the ideals I had about myself.

Now I have a primary purpose. It is founded upon the spiritual principles of the 12 Steps, such as honesty, humility, willingness, and courage, and the resulting goals of serenity and compassion. My dreams have taken on new meaning as I develop more and more self-confidence, and it all started with staying clean one day at a time. Quitting weed was just the first step. Now it is my responsibility to continue growing into a fuller expression of my spiritual recovery, empowerment, and freedom.

Final thought: Today, my primary purpose is to be of maximum service to my Higher Power and my fellows, especially the ones suffering from addiction.

August 26

Letting Go

"What we needed was a readiness to let go, and an openness to allow our loving God to do deep and lasting work in our hearts and minds."

- *Life With Hope*, first edition, page 25

Letting go does not always mean the obvious thing. Sometimes, letting go means allowing myself to feel rage. At other times, it means setting a boundary, and at other times still, it means sitting through pain. In recovery, I have learned to give myself permission to feel. Letting go allows me a space to navigate tough feelings. Sometimes, it is this opening that is integral to my process and journey of recovery. I am not perfect, nobody is, and it is a relief to know that there is no misunderstanding about that between me and God. My Higher Power is with me on this journey.

Final thought: Letting go for me today is rejoicing in the process, the acknowledgment that it is all going to be OK, and the comfort that I am human.

August 27

How Do You Know You're Addicted?

"At the end I was just smoking to stop the craving. Even though smoking pot wasn't fun, I couldn't stop"

- A Slave to Marijuana, Life with Hope, third edition, page 100

I started smoking "for fun" when I was 21. I eventually became a daily smoker—and eventually would have to push myself to not smoke before work. I was surrounded by people who believed and advocated that weed was a good thing. I was a pretty functional, moderately successful stoner. Everything seemed OK from my point of view—despite my emotional, social, and relational turmoil. When I was about 30 I wanted to quit and realized I couldn't. I found that it had power over me and that I was addicted. I figured if you want to quit something and can't, you're addicted. If you say "I don't want to do this" and within 24 hours (or sometimes minutes), you're doing it again, I'd say that's addiction. For seven years I tried to quit. Sometimes I'd be successful in going handfuls of months, and almost a year without it, but somehow I'd start again. I would be hooked again and would have to try to dig myself back out of addiction again.

Thank God for Marijuana Anonymous. I have had the most success in giving up weed, giving up alcohol, bettering my relationships, my behavior and my life through MA and the 12 Steps. I'm learning to recognize those feelings and triggers that previously made me want to smoke. I remember the many times when I smoked to relieve an emotion—only to have my emotional situation go the opposite way than I wanted. With the 12 Steps and MA, I'm finding healthy and more helpful ways to solve my problems—instead of numbing them down.

Final thought: God, help me to remember that if I smoke, weed will have total power over me again. I want to walk this recovery life with You and with my MA fellows.

August 28

Freedom From Shame and Guilt

"Our suffering shows us that we need to let go absolutely."

- How It Works, *Life With Hope*, third edition, page 193

I was a slave to marijuana. Pot chilled me out, but when I couldn't get high, I was aggressive, angry, and abusive to people I loved. I pushed people away and isolated myself. I used my so-called friends to keep getting high. I broke the law. I spent embarrassing amounts of money and time on getting pot, smoking pot, and avoiding anything that got in the way of getting high. I was hedonistic and selfish. When I first came to the rooms, I was filled with guilt and shame. I was convinced that I would be rejected for my behavior because I had rejected myself.

Fortunately, I found a sponsor and started to work the Steps and share my secrets. The more I opened up and continued to be welcomed back, the more I learned to trust others. Today, I don't just have freedom from my addiction to pot; I have freedom from the shame and guilt that overwhelmed me and kept me isolated from others. I have freedom from the "bondage of self." I still struggle with shame but I know that I have come a long way, even if I still have a lot to learn. If I can be grateful for the freedom recovery has given me, I can have hope that a little more freedom will shine through, if I am willing to work and wait.

Final thought: Today, I am grateful for how far I've come and I know I still have a long way to go.

August 29

Checking In

"Questioning and evaluating our actions and ourselves helps us to stay the 'right size.' "

- *Life with Hope*, first edition, page 52

In active addiction, I would often need to act immediately on a feeling or act impulsively. Now that I am sober, when difficult situations or feelings arise, it can be uncomfortable or confusing and my old ways of thinking may surface. In recovery I often need to pause to check in with my true motivations. I can take a moment to evaluate and ask myself, "Is this coming from love or fear? Is this my sober mind or my addict mind? Does this align with my Higher Power's will or my will?"

In these times, when I take a moment to check in, I can learn to not react from old thinking patterns. I can give myself the space and the time to consider the validity of my reactions and consider if I even need to take action.

Final thought: When I take time to check in and evaluate, I ensure that my motivations, my reactions and my decisions support my recovery and align with my Higher Power and my program.

August 30

All Are Welcome

"Our fellowship will always be safe if our main interest in attending MA meetings is to recover from addiction and help others recover as well."

- *Life With Hope*, second edition, page 82

People of every skin color, political affiliation, sexual preference, socio-economic status, and pre-existing health condition can be ensnared by marijuana addiction. It is a disease that transcends my independently held beliefs and values, as well as my social obligations and loyalties. My solution to the disease must also transcend my unrelated, situational positions in life. I must regard this foundational rule with reverence: that recovering and helping others to recover is the main interest in attending MA meetings. Relationships between fellows sometimes progress into friendships, romance, or heated rivalries. For example, I can think of one person in the program I feel animosity toward on a personal level. Despite my highly consistent contention, I am able to coexist in shared spaces because I am always willing to place recovery first.

Final thought: Today, I will remain stalwart in my devotion to keeping the Marijuana Anonymous rooms safe for people in recovery.

August 31

Stepping to Freedom

"Step One was the first step to freedom. We admitted our lack of power and our inability to control our lives."

- *Life with Hope*, third edition, page 5

Several times over the years, I had the thought that I was a marijuana addict. I would conveniently "forget" or minimize my struggle with weed. How could the substance that I believed took me to mystical heights, had cured my ills and was part of my identity, be a problem? It turns out marijuana wasn't magic or medicine! It had become madness and misery. I was always on some sort of self-improvement project but nothing worked for long. As life became more unmanageable, I began looking for answers.

One day, I came across Life with Hope and read Step One. Each sentence resonated in the core of my being. How did this book know so much about me and my life? It put words to what I had been feeling and experiencing. I wasn't alone. I wasn't any of the labels that I had shamefully assumed. I had a disease, the disease of addiction.

I repeated the phrase "I'm a marijuana addict" over and over. I said it at Marijuana Anonymous meetings. I wrote about it on my Step One. It unlocked a door I had been searching for my whole life.

Final thought: Today, I take another step to freedom by accepting my marijuana addiction, powerlessness, and unmanageability.

September 1

Amends—A Skillset Anyone Can Learn

"It is not the purpose of the Ninth Step to clear our conscience at the expense of others. We were careful not to have our amends adversely affect other people."

- Life with Hope, third edition, page 44

My first amends was to my mother, mostly for having expectations for her instead of accepting her as she was. Vulnerability felt awkward, so I prayed to God for sincerity. Afterward, I told my sponsor how my mother unexpectedly apologized back. I didn't know what to do. My sponsor told me that sometimes this happened, and I could express forgiveness back. My second amends was to my aunt for being a careless roommate. She said I didn't cause harm but was poor at communication. I wrote that down and agreed to make a living amends by changing my future behavior.

My third and fourth amends were to old roommates for erratic behavior. They forgave me and made excuses because I was young. I was careful to express gratitude for their compassion but still claim responsibility. I told my sponsor this, and she told me that sometimes people make excuses for us, and we can choose whether or not to accept them.

My fifth amends was to my stepmother whom my father had since divorced. We hadn't spoken in years. Our relationship started deteriorating when I started smoking pot at 14 because I was shameful and feared rejection. I shut her out. During the amends, I was careful with my speech because I had probably caused massive harm. I became acutely aware of her sensitivity and discerned when it was appropriate to save details for later rather than saying 'everything I needed to say.' I took responsibility but was careful to not cause more harm.

I have more amends to make. They were intimidating at first, but I learned something in each one and used these lessons to improve on the next. Like everything, even our amends are an opportunity for learning and making progress, not for perfection.

Final thought: Today, I make direct amends to such people wherever possible, except when to do so would injure them or others.

September 2

A Message to Higher Power

"God, grant me the serenity to accept the things I cannot change, the courage to change the things I can, and the wisdom to know the difference."

- Serenity Prayer, Life With Hope, third edition, page 199

Higher power, give me the will to keep going.

To live this life I live.

Even when times get hard, give me the strength and courage to strive again.

Higher power, I thank you for letting me be a child of yours.

I thank you for removing the darkness, and clouds from my mind.

For letting me have the light of life.

Higher power, I thank you for the new journey of life in sobriety.

Higher power, I thank you for letting me become myself again.

Final thought: Today, I am me again.

September 3

Spiritual Energy

"Once we admitted our powerlessness, we had to find a power greater than ourselves by which we could live."

- Life with Hope, second edition, page 5

It continues to bewilder me how a power greater than myself keeps me clean and sober. The electricity analogy helps when I remember that I don't know how electricity works, but I'm grateful it does when my heater keeps me warm on a cold day. My mind wants to understand this power greater than me while my heart wants me to relax and just be grateful that I'm no longer a slave to marijuana.

Before recovery, I didn't really know myself. I was moving through life in a cloud of smoke, every day like the last. Since working these Twelve Steps, I have come to know my values, my preferences, and my way of walking through the world. Recovery has given me the gift of faith, which I didn't know I needed or wanted, but which helps me trust in a power greater than myself, even if I don't understand it.

Final thought: Today, I trust my Higher Power cares for me and will help me stay clean if I do what is suggested.

September 4

Powerlessness

"Even though smoking pot wasn't fun, I couldn't stop. I've heard that one of the meanings of the word *addiction* is slavery, and I was truly a slave to marijuana."

- A Slave to Marijuana, Life with Hope, third edition, page 100

I am a marijuana addict. I always chuckled at the part we read that said, "Were you anxious when your stash was low?" My stash was never low. I was a functional addict, dealer, connoisseur, and purveyor of cannabis. My whole life and livelihood centered around it. If I were to run out, I would melt away like the Wicked Witch in the Wizard of Oz; that could never happen.

The sad part was that I never realized that subconsciously I dealt so that I would never run out. I had to always be numb. I couldn't possibly allow myself to feel emotions, people, and life. Through the MA program, I have come to learn that my life without weed has so much more to offer. I no longer live with anxiety every time I hear sirens or simply wake up. I have service positions and look forward to meetings as opposed to living hopelessly. I have friends who care about me legitimately, not because I am their source. I hope that soon I'll know peace.

Final thought: Today, I live a life with hope.

September 5

Following God's Will

"Step Nine allows us to practice all of the spiritual principles learned in the first eight steps..."

- *Life with Hope*, first edition, page 43

For many years, as a practicing addict, I was either above the universe or below it. I had great pride and great shame. This duality fueled my prideful and pitiful addiction. My pride told me that a world run on my will would make everything right. In recovery, I know that was nothing more than my EGO (Edging God Out). On the flip side, I had become so ashamed of my addiction and the turmoil it had caused in my life. The only method to assuage the pain was to use. Then, I would become ashamed I used, would use again to forget I was ashamed, and in turn the cycle would continue, round and round.

With recovery, I have learned that following the spiritual principles in our Steps has brought me to my Higher Power, whom I define as GOD (Good Orderly Direction). I understand today that I have a special place in the universe and a path to follow. This spiritual roadmap puts me into accordance with God's will, and following it provides serenity because I accept who I am, an addict in recovery, who follows the middle road of humility.

Final thought: Today, I will try to live my life, absent of pride and pity.

September 6

Living the Twelve Steps

"Practicing the principles we learn by taking the Twelve Steps produces rewards beyond calculation."

- Life with Hope, second edition, page 69

I found myself without direction. Upside-down and turned around, a marijuana addict merely existing and unable to solve life's challenges or issues in a healthy manner. All I had left were neurotic reactions. I had crossed the line. I was a marijuana junkie, a pothead monkey. I was tired of myself this way! "I need help! I want a life, I want to live!" I had gone it alone for 16 days when by the grace of a power greater than myself, I discovered the fellowship and a phone meeting of MA. At this point, nothing had changed except I wasn't using. It was suggested that I work the Twelve Steps with a sponsor, and so I did. I wanted change more than anything, I was willing to go to any lengths.

By working the Steps, I now had hope and began to learn and attain spiritual principles I could apply. By working the Twelve Steps, I transformed and had a personality change/psychic change, a spiritual awakening. Instead of using character defects, I have now shifted by responding to life and life's challenges and issues. I respond by applying the Twelve Steps; the spiritual principles of courage, humility, faith, integrity, to my life with positive results.

I live by the spiritual principles of recovery in all my affairs and under all conditions, to the best of my ability. I now have a purposeful meditative life. The obsession to smoke, smuggle, sell, buy, bake, eat, grow, and vape marijuana has been lifted. Everything has changed; recovery is my lifestyle, I have freedom to choose. I am grateful for a new way of life!

Final thought: Today, I am grateful.

September 7

Amends

"Wherever possible, we write down what we might do to set things straight with the people on our list."

- *MA Workbook*, first edition, 11th printing, page 44

Step Nine isn't just about saying I'm sorry, it is about an amend. What is an amend? It is the action of mending. We mend tears, repair them, heal them. Not all tears and wounds should be treated the same way; there isn't one specific way to make amends with everyone on my list. Surgeons have a variety of stitches and sutures depending on the wound. They will use the appropriate stitch to best support healing.

It is the same with amends. I think about an appropriate reparation. I found it helpful to put myself in the other person's shoes, to look at the harm from their perspective and ask myself, "what would it take to heal this? What could I say, or do, that will mend this tear?" While I don't know if it will heal the harm, I am considerate, thoughtful and mindful of my motives and actions. With this approach, I am repairing my attitude and demonstrating my changes.

In making amends, I take well-considered action. I practice the spiritual principles of the first nine Steps by being willing to be honest, hopeful, trusting in my Higher Power and this process, courageous to face those I have harmed, acting with integrity, being loving, forgiving, and doing what is just and fair.

Final thought: Today, I am able to act with integrity because I practice the spiritual principles of the Steps.

September 8

The Grace of God

"God has become a living force in our lives."

- Life with Hope, third edition, page 45

I was skeptical when I first was introduced to the Twelve Steps. Reference to God and a Higher Power made me leery and suspicious. Had it not been for permission to choose a version of God of my own understanding, I'm afraid that I may have remained trapped in my addiction. At first I used nature as evidence of a power greater than myself. Finally, I realized that I'm simply not capable of really understanding God. At the same time, I firmly believe in God. I don't have to understand God to believe in God. It's become abundantly clear that turning my will and my life over to this ambiguous Higher Power has set me free. Having the "obsession to use" lifted almost seems miraculous.

Final thought: Growing along spiritual lines continues to provide rewards "beyond calculation." I am forever grateful, to God, to the fellowship and the MA program for helping me to pursue the path of the Twelve Steps.

September 9

Perseverance, We Continue

"Each day we must do something to enhance our spiritual program. Our recovery depends on it."

- Life with Hope, first edition, page 50

I do not know God's will for me, it remains a beautiful mystery. I know that each and every day I can continue to open my heart, mind, and spirit to what that path is. In order to persevere in my recovery on a daily basis, I continue to ask for help and guidance from my Higher Power and mentors, turn my will over to the care and direction of God, and practice spiritual principles in all areas of my life.

I continue to have honest self-inquiry, humbly asking for the removal of my shortcomings, weed the garden, plant more seeds by which to grow spiritually, emotionally, and to work towards being the best person I can be. I disrupt patterns that no longer serve myself or others, admit when I am wrong, and am of service and help others to the best of my ability.

I long to be an instrument of peace and compassion, placing others before me, and doing what I can to alleviate suffering and cultivate happiness and love. I grow my spiritual practice through prayer, meditation, mantra, and practicing spiritual principles. I keep it simple, taking deep breaths, and let it go and give it to God.

I try to be present, open-minded, humble and teachable, to maintain a beginner's mind, practice gratitude, seek and practice new ways of spiritual development and study, and practice quieting my mind. I practice forgiveness, kindness and generosity, and keep asking for guidance. When intuitive answers come, listen, and have faith in the divine design of life.

I want always to have an open mind and hopeful heart, and remember that God loves me and wants me to be happy and fulfilled.

Final thought: I will continue to grow in my recovery, live in the sunlight of the spirit, and give away what continues to be so generously given to me.

September 10

Personal Recovery Depends Upon MA Unity

"We become willing to help our group deal constructively with conflict. As group members, we strive to work out difficulties openly, honestly, and fairly, and we seek to promote the common welfare of all members rather than a personal agenda. Each of us takes into consideration the effect our actions might have on newcomers."

- Life with Hope, third edition, page 66

In recovery, the experience I had as a newcomer can fade by the wayside as I become more confident in my recovery and more established in my group. It is not difficult to become a big fish in a little pond as more days are strung together. I must remember the adage that it is better to be kind than right when dealing with fellows, whether at a recovery meeting or a business meeting.

It is so important to try to keep in mind the perspective of a newcomer who isn't familiar with our jargon, slogans, and group dynamics and remember the sensitivity and fear that accompanied my own early days. Rather than avoiding conflict, I welcome the opportunity to grow up in the rooms, practicing how to resolve the inevitable difficulties that arise in any relationship, with the principles of the program. I may not always do it well or gracefully, but with patience, humility, and acceptance, I practice progress and growth while modeling it for others.

Final thought: Today, I will keep the newcomer in mind and put the unity of the fellowship on which my personal recovery depends first.

September 11

The Promises

"Miracles have become everyday reality...God has become a living force in our lives. We have grown free and joyful...Our attitude has turned from denial, defiance, and belligerence to gratitude, humility, and a sincere effort to be of service."

- Life with Hope, third edition, page 45

There were two things that made me want to come back to meetings when I was newly sober. People kept saying they had a life beyond their wildest dreams - a life without marijuana and with the Promises. Our literature is filled with Promises throughout every Step. The culmination of the Ninth Step Promises, as we know them, gave me so much hope. Today, I've worked the Twelve Steps and the Promises have come true for me too.

For nearly 20 years, I smoked weed all day, every day. Today, my life is unrecognizable and is beyond anything I could have dreamed of while in active addiction. I didn't hit the jackpot, quit my job, and buy a private island. I don't have to, in order to experience a life beyond my wildest dreams. I have seen everyday miracles, starting with the fact that I don't need to wake and bake the second my alarm goes off.

I am connected with a positive Higher Power that loves me and wants the best for me. I have experienced joy in ways I never thought possible; a way that no amount of marijuana ever brought into my life. Each day, I'm filled with gratitude and awe. This life is a valuable gift, one that I don't take for granted. To keep it, I continue to work my own program, and help other marijuana addicts with theirs.

Final thought: Today, I will say thank you to my Higher Power and Marijuana Anonymous for a life beyond my wildest dreams.

September 12

Connection

"I spent most of my time with my using friends, who became my closest network."

- I Found MA Online, *Life with Hope*, second edition, page 140

During my using career, I have cycled through many groups of friends. Many of them used marijuana. I only gravitated toward others who used. Fast forward to the present moment; not a single one of them is still in my life today. Marijuana was the only glue that bound me to them. To think that these individuals were my closest network of friends is a complete tragedy. None of them stood by me when I hit my rock bottom and became homeless, jobless, hopeless, and helpless. This is the life of marijuana addiction; fickle friendships and loneliness.

On the other end of the spectrum is recovery and hope. Hanging out on this end, I have formed and cultivated meaningful relationships with others in the program. I have met a handful of other recovering addicts who have become close friends; people who I can count on to support me, lift me up, and have my back during difficult times. I also have my sponsor to lean on, and I have sponsees with whom I've built deep connections; what beautiful gifts of sobriety! Meaningful connections with others in the program have kept me clean, resilient, and joyful. My life has an added dimension of community through fellowship and connection. I no longer feel lonely. With the help of the MA fellowship, I feel safe, respected, and whole.

Final thought: Today, I build meaningful relationships by connecting with others in the program.

September 13

Take a Look in the Mirror First

"We made amends even to those who had harmed us more than we had harmed them, regardless of whether they reciprocated."

- *Life with Hope*, third edition, page 44

I had enough resentments to fill a swimming pool and just floated in them until I became all withered and soggy. I hung on to those because they justified my anger and made me feel superior to those who I felt had wronged me. I remember doing my first Fourth Step inventory and I kept saying, "but they…" My sponsor stopped me and said, "this inventory is not about them, it is about you and what you did. You have to take care of your side of the street."

It was humbling to let go of those resentments and look at what I had done in those relationships. I realized that to fix this, I had to make the amends for what I had done without mentioning the resentments and the wrongs that I felt were done to me. Once I was willing to discuss only my part, I found that I was able to mend many of the relationships that had gone wrong. Also I found that some of them were willing to take on their part in the situation and we could move forward as better friends.

Final thought: Today, I accept that my life is the way that it is because of the choices I have made, and I must be willing to take responsibility for what I do and say.

September 14

Counting My Blessings

"All we need is to maintain an open mind and a hopeful heart."

- Life with Hope, second edition, page 7

I like making gratitude lists. Sometimes it's hard for me to focus on the positive, while it's so easy to be negative. But just jotting down a couple things I'm grateful for really helps me change my perspective and attitude.

If I'm really having a tough time, sometimes all I can do is be grateful for the fact that I'm alive, and able to have emotions. Positive or negative, whether I feel numb or overstimulated. I try to embrace the ebb and flow of life.

Also I've come to a place in recovery where I'm learning to be grateful for the negative things I've been through: trauma, abuse, etc. Because I wouldn't be where I am, who I am, today without having gone through those hardships. It seems strange to be grateful for bad things having happened, but this is my soul journey. I am meant to learn from and overcome the obstacles my higher power places in front of me.

Today, I choose to do my best to tap into positive energy. There are positive and negative energies all around me in recovery every day. Today, I will do my best to tap into the positive. I can start right now by counting my blessings.

Final thought: Higher Power, thank you for the blessings I have received in my recovery.

September 15

One Day at a Time

"Our message is one of hope and promise that any addict can stop using marijuana, lose the obsession and desire to do so, and find a new way of life by following spiritual principles one day at a time."

- Life with Hope, second edition, page 82

This message, as part of Tradition Five, is the golden goose of recovery. The thought of staying clean for a lifetime would weigh me down and feel heavy on my heart, but through the practice of taking the program just one day at a time, the weight of recovery is lifted. The pressure to stay clean becomes more manageable, easier to handle, and downright doable. I also used to think that I would never be able to stop using marijuana and would continue to drown in obsessive thoughts of using for the rest of my life. I thought there was no hope for me and that I'd be an addict for life. I didn't think there was any possibility for me to stay clean, because I thought I was different.

In all actuality, I fit right in with my fellow addicts in recovery. I have been navigating this new territory called "A Clean Life," and all I had to do was to follow a set of principles outlined in the 12 Steps of recovery, leading me toward my spiritual awakenings and long-term sobriety. The most important piece to it all is ODAAT, "One Day At A Time." There is hope in these rooms. There is hope for each and every one of us who struggles with marijuana addiction. We can live a life with hope—one day at a time.

Final thought: Today, I practice the principles of the program one day at a time.

September 16

Potential

"We were living the fantasy of functionality."

- *Life with Hope*, second edition, page 2

Before I started recovery I considered myself a "functional stoner." I would go to work high every day, I would drive high, I even went to job interviews high because that's how I would be on the job. I never really realized that I was only functioning at a bare minimum. All I did was go to work and go home and all I did in between was smoke weed.

Once I got clean, I had all this energy and drive to do more. I would hang out with friends, I started climbing and swimming again. I even decided to go back to school and finally finish that degree that I gave up on when I first started smoking because "I wasn't sure what I wanted to do." Getting clean has been the greatest thing for me because I now know that I have this amazing potential that I can live up to. My life isn't just getting high and working the same stupid job every day.

Final thought: Today, I will work towards my goals of living up to my full potential.

September 17

Identity

"It seemed so right at the time. Smoking pot was a way of declaring my independence and establishing an identity."

- A Life Worth Living, *Life with Hope*, second edition, page 165

Throughout my life, my identity was very much defined by smoking herbs. However, the day came when I realized that I was addicted and I felt a new identity emerge, one based on who I truly am and not anchored in some substance. From the realization that I was not a person because of drugs, but rather from being a person in myself, set me free to pursue a larger I, and with the help from my new family, a greater We. Today, I stand as a human who has discovered many layers of self that were not available to me while numbing my conscious and unconscious self with marijuana.

Final thought: Today, I am thankful for being a fuller and more present human being.

September 18

The Twelve Questions

"Do you smoke pot to cope with your feelings?"

- The Twelve Questions, *Life with Hope*, third edition, page 192

When I came to MA and heard the Twelve Questions read aloud, Question Six jumped out at me. I had been raised in an abusive, alcoholic home and my feelings were on red alert all the time. I had developed a cool, "who cares?" attitude by the age of six. I wasn't going to be believed, much less protected. I felt like it was a dog-eat-dog world and I would get mine any way I could. This attitude alternated with my sensitive side, which marveled at nature's wonders and yearned for a spiritual connection. Being a hero or a martyr changed with my outlaw rebelliousness on a daily basis.

As I grew, I knew my feelings were far too intense; but I thought it was my "artistic temperament" or just being a misfit. When I discovered pot, it was magical. I wasn't angry or anxious. "Sad" and "mad" were the only feelings I could identify, and now I could just stay high. This honeymoon phase was quickly followed by dropping out of school, alienating family and friends, and becoming totally unreliable.

In the program, I learned feelings aren't facts! I could deal with a mistake or a hurt—an "oops" or an "ouch" as a sponsor put it—without having to use. This was incredibly freeing, but it did not happen overnight. Even now, when I feel something intensely, I have tools to use and a God to thank.

Final thought: Today, I will allow my loving God to do deep and lasting work in my heart and mind.

September 19

Willingness to Try Again

"The turning point for us was the decision to relinquish control. However, no matter how sincere our efforts, we do make mistakes. Then we admit our humanity and try again."

- *Life with Hope*, first edition, page 14

In my early twenties, I was an active member in meeting rooms. I was able to maintain a few years of abstinence, but there was still much about the Twelve Steps I never fully understood. I resisted applying certain concepts to my recovery. I thought I had "completed" all the work and could just stop engaging with my recovery process. I forgot that I am powerless to manage my addiction, and once again I tried to control my use. All my previous gains of recovery went dormant as my life became increasingly unmanageable and my disease progressed to new levels of destruction. I became desperate for help, emotionally distraught, and I had no idea what to do.

Now in my mid-thirties, I found the humility to return to meetings. This time, I'm embracing recovery as if I were drowning and grabbing onto a life preserver. The gift of desperation made me open to finally surrendering to forces much greater than my ego. Not knowing what to do has opened me to receiving guidance from others, and given me a willingness to try a different way of being.

I am now actively applying the Steps to my life and letting go of the underlying trauma and fears that kept me using. I believe there is a possibility for healing the moment we begin to trust the unfolding process. I know I am powerless over marijuana. I reach out for help rather than always running away from myself. It is not always easy, but it is far more sustainable than my life of using. Now, I have a second chance to experience myself, other people, and my concept of Higher Powers in a new way.

Final thought: Today, I turn my desperation into a willingness to reach out for help. I have trust in this process.

September 20

Our Mission

"The story of the Lotus Eaters speaks particularly to us dopeheads. As addicts, we were stuck in a Lotus Land; we forgot our mission; we forgot the other adventures that awaited us; we forgot about going home."

- Life with Hope, third edition, page xxi

When I first read the story of the Lotus Eaters I was struggling with letting go of marijuana. I was stuck in a "Lotus Land." I cried every time I used, wondering if this would ever stop. In the process of my addiction I did forget what my mission was. I forgot about all of life's adventures that waited for me. I didn't know how to get out. All I knew at the time was that I needed to keep coming to Marijuana Anonymous meetings to help me figure it out.

As I kept attending, I was discovering more about myself. I was discovering more about my Higher Power. I channeled this and soon discovered I too was like the scouts on my journey, again rowing like hell. I don't know where I'm going next. I'm just trying to stay clean today; maybe that's my mission for now.

Final thought: I don't know where tomorrow will take me, but I do know that today I will be clean

September 21

Our Will vs. God's Will

"Our inability to surrender had always blocked the effective entry of a Higher Power into our lives."

- Life with Hope, third edition, page 11

When I gave up my insistence to enforce my will in every single thing I did, or thought I should do, and instead asked God's will to guide my life, I was able to surrender. It was hard at first because I thought I was driving the universe with my every thought and action. When I realized I was not in control, and could ask for God's will and guidance, life became easier to take. I was less stressed and looked less at tomorrow and lived more for today.

It is hard at first, don't get me wrong. When I live in the will, grace, and guidance of the Creator, and do not expect anything, I can concentrate more on my next step and not 1,000 steps down the line. The next step becomes more clear, the next right thing is more apparent. Avoiding a mistake, like smoking a joint because I am stressed out or angry, became more second nature to me. I was able to say, "hey, what did I learn from this?" or, "what should I do next?" I have increasingly been able to make good decisions and not stew in self-pity and resentment of others.

Final thought: Today, I will walk by faith, not by sight.

September 22

Compassion Instead of Denial

"We stopped practicing denial and became willing to face our disease."

- *Life with Hope*, first edition, page 3

The other day, I was watching a guy take some hits off a pipe inside his car. He didn't move or change his gaze from a blank stare for almost a minute. I don't think he was aware of me watching him even though I was less than ten feet away. The overwhelming feeling I felt in that instant was one of compassion, a compassion that hoped he could eventually find the strength to put the bong down. I couldn't help but remember all of the times when I was in his position. I remembered the sensation of basically having my brain fall asleep while the rest of me was still awake, something a non-pothead can't understand but every pothead knows all too well.

As I sat there, I realized I was having an out-of-body experience, but in a much different way than I did when I was still smoking. This time the out-of-body experience was me putting myself in someone else's shoes. I had never done this when I was getting high because I was too worried about making myself feel good to care or even think about how anyone else was feeling.

In times when life on life's terms seems to be getting the best of me, I remember where I came from before entering recovery. This gives me a new perspective and helps me to see that what I had seen as major problems were really insignificant or, even blessings, in some cases. I don't punish myself when recalling these situations that I never want to live again but instead choose to remember and recognize the difference between where I took myself then and where God is taking me now.

Final thought: For today, I ask myself, "What would happen if I allowed myself to see the world as others see it? What kind of understanding would I gain?"

September 23

Humility

"...recovery from addiction requires resources beyond the capacities of any one individual addict."

- Life with Hope, first edition, page 8

In recovery, I often hear about acceptance and how this leads to serenity but how I do this is much more of a challenge. The process of working the Steps helps to put my life into perspective by understanding my limitations. I am not the best or the worst person in the world. The grandiosity that fuels the extremes of inflation and deflation are ego-based. The Steps help me be right-sized, knowing my strengths and weaknesses.

When I learn humility by this process, I can feel the grace and dignity that comes with using intelligent spiritual action to deal with my problems. Not having to rely on my limited personal experience filled with anxiety, but rather on the collected wisdom of recovery, takes away the pressure to do it alone.

With help and support, the gifts of working a recovery program, my life becomes serene, based on a spiritual connection with our Higher Power. When I am able to follow the guidance of my Higher Power, my life has meaning, purpose, and serenity.

Final thought: Today, I live my life by accepting who I am because I know that I am not perfect.

September 24

Let Go and Let God

"Petty problems have stopped bedeviling us."

- Life with Hope, third edition, page 45

I was an expert at getting bent out of shape by problems that I encountered in my daily life. It didn't take much for me to get disturbed by things that didn't line up with my view of what should and shouldn't be. It didn't take much for me to get my nose out of joint, become angry, or feel sorry for myself. Constantly assigning my view of what should or shouldn't be, caused me needless angst and was totally useless. The real problem was me, not what was or wasn't going on in my daily life. My unrealistic and selfish expectations led me to be easily disappointed or disturbed. Turning my will and life over to the care of God has helped me to let go and "go with the flow."

Final thought: I live in peace when I "let go and let God."

September 25

Toolkits

"We now have tools to help us grow."

- *Life with Hope*, second edition, page 63

I've heard people talk in meetings about recovery giving them a spiritual toolkit. I access these tools as needed to help me continue on the path of being and staying clean. My spiritual toolkit includes meetings, working the Steps, calling my sponsor or a friend in recovery, and practicing prayer and meditation. It also includes the slogans, affirmations, and learning to focus on my physical well-being as well as my mental, spiritual, and emotional health.

I recently heard something new: that our disease of addiction has a toolkit too! Actually, it's more like a cache of weapons! It contains things like fear, shame, guilt, pride, and making comparisons. Now, when those thoughts creep in, I remember they are part of my addiction, and I turn to my recovery toolkit to handle them. I remember that comparing my insides to another's outside is never helpful. When I feel shame or guilt, I try to remember to call someone to talk it through so I can move through those feelings. I know that pain is inevitable, but that suffering is optional. With my spiritual toolkit, I can relieve my unnecessary suffering much quicker than before recovery.

Final thought: Today, I go through my day with my spiritual toolkit always ready by my side.

September 26

The Opposite of Addiction Is Connection

"It was a best friend for years and then it turned on us."

- Life with Hope, third edition, page 4

When I first started smoking cannabis, it was to cope with the side effects of autoimmune disease and chemotherapy. I was always a studious type of kid who was never going to use drugs. When I was sick and missing class, a friend offered it to me to help with nausea and pain. At first, it was helpful and I only used it when sickness kept me from going to class. Slowly it became the coping mechanism for every difficulty I encountered in my life. When I was sexually assaulted, I started smoking every day. It allowed me to block out some of that pain and cope with the fact that I was in an abusive relationship. I thought that cannabis allowed me to endure my struggles, when really it kept me from confronting them and improving my life.

After my best friend took her life, I was smoking from the moment I woke up until I fell asleep. I had lost my closest friend, but instead of seeking comfort or companionship from others, I sat locked away in my room completely alone. I did not realize that cannabis had caused me to withdraw from others into my own isolated world. I spent my days stoned and alone, trying to repress my thoughts and feelings.

When I joined Marijuana Anonymous I not only gained sobriety, but rooms full of supportive people who encouraged me to share my feelings. I learned to leave my own personal bubble and rejoin the land of the living. Now, I have a group of supportive and clean friends with whom I am so excited to talk and share each day.

Final thought: Now, my life is filled with genuine human connection instead of the isolation of addiction.

September 27

The Gifts of the Program

"The rewards we've received...are profound and sublime."

- Life with Hope, third edition, page 45

After years of smoking pot, I was trapped in addiction. I continually caved to the ongoing cravings that crept up throughout the day and night. I was smoking around the clock. I had become powerless and needless to say, my life had become unmanageable.

I was desperate and was relieved to learn about Marijuana Anonymous. I came to believe that if I joined the MA fellowship, turned my will and life over to the care of God, (even though I didn't understand God), worked the Steps and practiced the principles of the program, I could be set free from the bondage of my addiction. I had been told to attend "ninety meetings in ninety days," but I ended up attending more than one meeting a day at the beginning of my recovery.

I was more than willing to trade the captivity of my addiction for freedom from addiction. What I have found as I've followed the path of the Twelve Steps are "rewards beyond calculation.

Final thought: I will be forever grateful for the innumerable gifts that I've received from the MA program.

September 28

Higher Power Connection

"Although many of us came to the fellowship already believing in the existence of a Higher Power, we doubted that it would be of help since it had not helped us to stay clean before."

- Life with Hope, third edition, page 9

In the beginning of my recovery, I attempted to cast aside my atheism to allow religious versions of God into my heart. This was not entirely effective for me. I was desperate enough, so I tried my hardest to surrender. I associated this version of a Higher Power with certain strictures, ways of thinking, and standards of conduct that my nature profoundly resisted. It was indeed a Higher Power, but it was not my Higher Power.

As I continued attending meetings and working the Steps, I came to understand better. My sponsor put it best, telling me that my Higher Power can be anything as long as it loves you unconditionally and it's greater than you are. He also explained that my connection with my Higher Power could evolve over time. When I was allowed to conceive of my Higher Power in a less paternally prescribed manner, I found my connection with my Higher Power became far stronger.

I know now that my Higher Power wants for me the very best of what I want for myself. Now, I pray twice every day. Once in the morning, I say, "Dear God, please help me gracefully follow your path today." Once in the evening, I say, "Dear God, today was a good day. Thank you for helping me hold to my values. I love you." As I continue to live in harmony with my Higher Power's will for me, I find my feeling of connection grows steadily, and I see my life continue to improve.

Final thought: Today promises to be a good day, as I live it holding to my values by the grace of my Higher Power.

September 29

No More Doom and Gloom

"Our awakening has come about as a result of a spiritual house cleaning, being aware of who we are, and cultivating a growing relationship with our Higher Power."

- *Life with Hope*, second edition, page 68

Once I got clean, and the fog of marijuana left my body, mind and spirit, I realized that for me a large part of being addicted meant focusing on the negative. I was never exposed to the concept of gratitude until I went to 12-Step meetings. Focusing on what's wrong was a lifelong habit, but one I wanted to break. Similar to how I don't want marijuana to steal one more day from me, I likewise don't want doom and gloom to crowd my day. I choose joy today. I choose to focus on what's working in my life. Fortunately, I have the Twelve Steps to resolve old resentments and grief.

Marijuana had kept me prisoner for half my life when I was finally able to accept the grace that life offered and I entered recovery. I had no idea what was in store for me: learning who I am; what I value; and how my past had affected me. I learned I had choices, and that I could choose to stay clean, if I could do it one day at a time. There was a person celebrating five years in my first meeting, and I found that impossible to believe. I could not imagine going one week without pot, but the next day I didn't smoke pot, and I haven't since then. I'm grateful for the wonderful life I have today, and all the blessings recovery has brought me.

Final thought: Today, I choose to focus on what's right, and stay away from focusing on what's wrong.

September 30

Cleaning Up The Wreckage of the Past

"Step Nine allows us to practice all of the spiritual principles encompassed in the first eight steps, with the addition of the principle of justice."

- Life with Hope, first edition, page 43

The Ninth Step is a series of actions I took in order to complete the work or process I began in Step Four, to clean up the wreckage of my past. Empowered with an inventory of my resentments and fears, I could now go further to make amends to those whom I had caused suffering. Sometimes a simple apology was not possible, but it was always possible to make a living amends through right action. Donating time at institutions, sending out literature to the addict who still suffers, taking a service position in MA are some examples of living amends. Turning it over and talking to my sponsor beforehand gave me the courage to face people I needed to speak with.

Final thought: Today, I will remember that I can make amends in many different ways.

October 1

Step Ten

"Each day, we renew our commitment to spiritual progress in order to stay one step ahead of the progressive disease of addiction"

- Life with Hope, first edition, page 49

When I act on defects, when life presents challenges, when my body becomes injured or ill, it's an opportunity to grow and learn. I can learn about love, learn about forgiveness, learn about acceptance or present moment awareness. Yet, sometimes I become worried about growing or progressing enough. It's a paradox of the spiritual path; knowing there's perfection in my imperfection. Right here, right now, deep down, there's a place of wholeness. On the flip side, I strive for progress in my dedication to my practices, guided by my desire to continue evolving into the next best version of myself. When I dedicate myself to my recovery process—the combination of "improving our conscious contact with God" and the reflection of "continuing to take personal inventory"—my growth and learning happen as natural outcomes.

Final thought: When I have faith in this process it leads me to where I am meant to go.

October 2

Strength in Faith

"Step Three was a decision not only to have faith but also to live by faith."

- *Life with Hope*, first edition, page 13

Sometimes I feel like, "Why me? Why does this stuff happen to me?" I know that the experiences I go through only help me become a stronger, better person. I learn through my experiences. I have to go through these times of trials and tribulations just to get to the point that I am trying to reach. A life of addiction is a life of self-centeredness. My needs became foremost in my priorities; I needed my drugs, my satisfactions, and my way in all things. The loudest voice I heard was the one in my head.

I took Step Three with my sponsor, and I learned how to "turn it over" and to "let go and let God." I heard these sayings at MA meetings and I was able to apply these to my recovery. My growth and recovery blossomed after I learned to trust my Higher Power. It was a relief to give up control. I am happy to have faith and acceptance as solutions to my problems.

Making a decision to turn my life over to my Higher Power was necessary for my recovery. In recovery I learned to wait, to become open to surrendering my will and life to a power greater than myself. I learned to put my needs aside and actively help others.

Final thought: I have strength in my faith to get through any situation.

October 3

Honesty

"This is a matter of self-preservation..."

- Life with Hope, first edition, page 53

There are two inventories in our 12-Step program and each is about honesty. The Fourth Step was an honest admission of our fearless moral inventory and the beginning of the action steps. In the Tenth Step, we continued to take personal inventory and when we were wrong, promptly admitted it. We continued to ask for more awareness and help in Marijuana Anonymous and our assets and liabilities require a spot-check.

My sponsor described this to me as, "shooting an arrow towards a target." Was I aiming in the right direction, close to the target or hitting the bulls-eye? Self-preservation was an action of maintaining and preserving what I started. I stopped using, lost the desire to use marijuana, and I was now finding a new life without marijuana in all its forms.

I remain vigilant from being complacent. I attend meetings, work with newcomers, and grow spiritually. As I become more open and willing, my inventory will promptly inform me when I am wrong. This is an ego-deflation exercise, but essential for me to grow and to handle conflict in a healthy constructive way.

Final thought: Today, the Steps maintain my preservation of this new life free of marijuana.

October 4

Humility

"The humility of asking for help keeps us from self-righteousness and protects us against outbreaks of either grandiosity or self-pity."

- Life with Hope, first edition, page 51

As I continue my path in recovery, I still occasionally experience flare-ups of ego and willfulness. It can happen anywhere: when I'm around family, while I'm driving, or at work. If I'm not paying attention to where my mind is wandering, my thoughts can take control of me and convince me that my old ways of thinking—that the world is working against me, that I'm in this alone—are fact.

At the end of the day, I sit down for a daily inventory and ask myself things like, "did I talk to my sponsor today?" and "was I overly emotional?" Yes, it is embarrassing when I tell my sponsor I let myself get so angry that I slammed my hand down on a table or that I flipped off another driver. With several years of sobriety, I'm supposed to have full control of myself by now! It is significant that today I have help from others with whom I can work, who give me proper perspective on my thoughts and actions. No longer do I need to get through life on my own.

Final thought: With pride, there are many curses. Today, I remember that with humility, there come many blessings.

October 5

Choose Your "Hard"

"Our program is not easy, but it is simple."

- How It Works, *Life with Hope*, third edition, page 193

Working the Twelve Steps of Marijuana Anonymous is hard work. The following things are also hard work: experiencing withdrawals from weed; feeling my feelings without the pacifier of pot to cover them up; showing up at meetings, sharing at meetings; talking to other humans, trusting other humans; the idea of a Higher Power, trusting that Higher Power; healing a lifetime of grief, resentments and fears; forgiving myself, admitting my faults; and changing every aspect of my life is hard work.

Living in active marijuana addiction is hard work: smoking weed all day, every day; saying no to people, places, and things that got in the way of smoking weed; not knowing who I am without marijuana; not wanting to know who I am without marijuana; hiding and sneaking around; avoiding humans, avoiding my feelings, avoiding my responsibilities; being angry at God; settling for less than I deserve, surviving paycheck to paycheck, living under a mountain of debt; burying a lifetime of grief, resentments, and fears; hating myself, hating the idea of one more day is hard work.

Which "hard" would I rather have? With the help of the Twelve Steps and my Higher Power, I've been given a beautiful life that I never thought was possible. I choose the hard work of living in recovery, rather than going back to the hard, hopeless, empty way I lived for nearly 20 years of active addiction.

Thank you Marijuana Anonymous, and thank you Higher Power.

Final thought: Today, I will choose the hard work of living in recovery and will see the promises fulfilled in my life.

October 6

Grace

"Our common welfare should come first; personal recovery depends on MA unity."

- *Life with Hope*, first edition, page 73

Grace is not just what you do at dinner before you eat, it's a gift. One definition of grace is a kindness extended to someone who doesn't deserve it. For a long time I never really understood what grace was, its true definition eluded me. When I got clean and had been attending meetings for a few months, eventually the veil was lifted and I finally got to understand grace by experiencing it first-hand. A kindness had been extended to me and I know I did nothing to deserve it.

I remember packing a pipe going down the freeway at 75 miles an hour; I could have had a very different bottom than the one that I had. I did a lot of things that were risky and stupid. I was led to the program of MA, and that is truly grace; for that I am grateful.

Final thought: Every day, I can count the many kindnesses extended to me, I could count them to the end of my days. Thank you, Higher Power for your grace and watching out for me.

October 7

God, As We Understood God

"Step Three: *Made a decision to turn our will and our lives over to the care of God, <u>as we understood God</u>.*"

- *Life with Hope*, first edition, page 11

God, mentioned eight times in the Twelve Steps, is a big part of our program. I am most fascinated by the concept of "*...God, as we understood God.*" I grew up in an evangelical Pentecostal church in the South. While that may work for many, it did not work for me. I was afraid of that God. My insides did not match up with that God; in short, I did not understand that God. For the Twelve Steps to work, I must exist and work within a concept of a God that I can understand.

The Twelve Steps give me permission to go with what I feel on the inside, as opposed to trying to make myself live up to a thought system that does not mesh with my own instincts. In a way, I'm grateful for my addiction; it got me into the rooms where I was given permission to trust my own understanding of a Higher Power.

Final thought: Today, I give thanks for my Higher Power. I have been given permission by the Twelve Steps to trust my own spiritual intuition.

October 8

Response + Ability = Responsibility

"As we grow in love and understanding, we gain an ability to reach out beyond ourselves."

- Life with Hope, first edition, page 61

Responsibility always seemed like a tremendous burden to me when I was using, something heavy and arduous like discipline or commitment—both of which felt overwhelming. It wasn't until I'd been clean for a few years that I began to cherish my "ability to respond" which means, for me now, the ability to show up (often on time!) and do what needs to be done. This includes the basics like: sleeping when I am tired, eating when I am hungry, and calling someone when I am lonely. It also includes the more complex tasks of making and keeping good boundaries. I have learned that "response-ability" is about being present, dealing with what is here-and-now rather than anguishing over past mistakes or future tripping.

Final thought: Today, "response-ability" allows me to be a person of integrity: caring and compassionate for others while at the same time staying aligned with my own goals, needs and values.

October 9

Remember to Surrender

"Our inability to surrender had always blocked the effective entry of a Higher Power into our lives."

- Life with Hope, first edition, page 11

Surrender is:

> The sweet bliss of letting go...and letting God,

> What I remember when I'm in a lot of pain,

> Usually my last resort,

> The result of practicing the Third Step,

> Something I need to practice over, and over, and over.

The first time I practiced a formal Third Step was the first time I surrendered. I was in my first year of recovery and I honestly believed I would only have to do the Third Step once. The feeling of surrender was much better than getting high, and I thought that I had found nirvana, that I would be happy and serene for the rest of my life.

Then life happened; I woke up the next day and had to do it again! This was the beginning of learning discipline, that awful word I had hated before recovery, but which has become an important part of my recovery. I need to practice the principles of this program every day. Daily practice takes discipline. I've learned that life is much easier if I do a Third Step every day (or even more often). I offer my will and my life to my Higher Power every day and ask to be shown what I should do.

When I surrender, I acknowledge that I'm not in charge. I know that I am happier and more serene when I let go of needing to be in charge, and I learn to trust in my Higher Power's will for me. Through daily effort, I come closer to understanding what my Higher Power wants to reveal to me.

Final thought: I offer my will and my life to my Higher Power every day and ask to be shown what I should do.

October 10

Can There Be Physical Effects from Quitting Marijuana?

"In spite of the common belief that there are no physiological or psychological effects of cannabis/marijuana addiction, a large number of recovering MA members experience withdrawal symptoms in some form as they stop using marijuana."

- *About Marijuana Detox*, MA pamphlet

Withdrawal symptoms are very real for many marijuana addicts. Withdrawal from marijuana, until recently, was considered non-existent. In talking with other marijuana addicts, I have found a different belief. They shared with me about their experience of having sleepless nights, night sweats, and an array of other symptoms. For me, withdrawal manifested itself in loss of appetite and crazy dreams. Extreme fatigue also reared its pull on me in early recovery. Now that I have detoxed from weed, my mind has cleared up, my thoughts are not so self-centered, and I am finding a new connection to my highest power.

Final thought: Today, I am so grateful I have gotten through my detoxing from marijuana. I am here to share that it does get better, one day at a time.

October 11

The Gift of Forgiveness

"We did this even though we may have not felt forgiving. The feeling of forgiveness may come some time after the act of forgiving."

- *Life with Hope*, third edition, page 38

Holding on to my resentments slowly consumed my spirit. I formed bricks with each one and stacked them between myself and others. I became convinced that connection only brought pain. I waited for sincere apologies from those who had deeply harmed me. The longer I waited, the longer the hurt remained. Recovery allowed me to see that the holding on was the problem. I was never going to hear what I had hoped; however, it was in my power to release this burden of hate.

Quietly, to myself, I vowed to let these resentments go. At first it didn't sit well with me. It didn't feel right after attaching myself to these feelings for so long. As I turned my focus inward and examined the ways that I had contributed to these situations, I began to realize it wasn't always as black and white as I thought. There was so much gray space to consider. In time, I forgave every person that had hurt me. I began to see their humanity. Their pain had caused them to pass it along to someone else. I knew it had to stop with me. This didn't mean that I had to allow them all back into my life or to forget what had happened between us.

Instead, I opened myself up to healthy connections knowing they were a necessary component to healing. I learned to create boundaries that allowed me to trust people again while also keeping myself safe. I have faith that this shift in perspective will bring me more joy and contentment than I have ever experienced before.

Final thought: Just for today, I will practice the act of forgiveness even if I don't feel ready. I have faith that it will feel more genuine in time.

October 12

Trust

"The Third Step does *not* say, 'We turned our will and our lives over to the care of God, *as we understood God.*' It says rather, 'We made a decision to do so.' "

- Life with Hope, second edition, page 12

I was told I was a willful child and that I made my own decisions. I was also told, "you're smart, but don't be stupid." With adults undermining me, I felt I could not trust anyone, and so I never felt connected to my Higher Power. I questioned myself constantly.

When taking the Third Step and making a decision to turn over my life to my Higher Power, I realized this is a daily and sometimes moment-to-moment decision. It's almost like doing a Tenth Step in a different way; taking inventory of what I have yet to release and deciding to do so. When I hold on so tightly that I can feel my nails digging into my palms, I have to let go, absolutely. I pray to let go of my will and follow God's will.

Each time I let go, it has turned out for the better. When I let go and pray, I can feel the belief and trust in me grow. Trust has always been hard for me (growing up in an abusive home) but trust feels so warm and comforting now. I love to trust myself, others and my Higher Power. It feels like I am on the right path; even though the facts of my life have not changed, my outlook on those facts has.

Final thought: Today, I am better each moment I let go and let God. I feel the change in my bones; I am in recovery; and I am a more serene person because of that decision.

October 13

Progressing in the Program

"We learn to give without expecting rewards. We act as responsible members of society, living not in isolation but with a sense of community."

- *Life with Hope*, first edition, page 68

For so long, I got high and isolated. I felt unlovable and worthless. Eventually, I realized that I didn't want marijuana in my life; I didn't want depression and isolation. When I came into MA I found that I didn't have to live this way. I found love and understanding. I know that my disease of marijuana addiction is progressive and know that my recovery can be progressive too.

In recovery, I have the things that I always wanted: love, connection to my Higher Power, and acceptance. I am grateful that I can enjoy life every day. I can participate in my life now, instead of watching life pass me by. Recovery helps me to be my true self. I can love myself and let others love me. I work at loving myself and I will work just as hard as I have at not liking myself. Now I ask my Higher Power for guidance so that I can try to do the next right thing with joy. I know that my Higher Power's plan will always result in the highest possible good. Now I can live a life of serenity, honesty, and joy, while staying present and being of service to others, one day at a time.

Final thought: Every day, I thank my Higher Power for another day, clean and sober. I ask my Higher Power for the knowledge that I'm lovable and capable of giving and receiving love.

October 14

Turning Over a Place

"To reopen old wounds that we may have felt were largely healed may seem pointless and painful, but we found that this process was essential to our new life and our new beginning."

- Life with Hope, third edition, page 36

When I was using, I had my favorite places I would associate with using marijuana. I have found it helpful to go back to those places and transform them into a clean serene environment. I call this "turning over a place." I like to go back to those places and instead of getting high I will now read a book, eat something healthy, or silently sit and observe the glory that is Higher Power.

For some of us, the places might actually be activities, which is OK, then I "turn over" picking up the kids, or attending a business meeting, or going shopping. The first place that I turned over was the cabinet above my stove. It used to be filled with paraphernalia and copious amounts of marijuana. Shortly after becoming clean I cleared out that cabinet and filled it with rice, beans, oatmeal, berries, and the like. Immediately following this action I found my cravings drastically reduced. Now, quite frequently when I open that cabinet, I feel calm and a comforting joy.

Final thought: For today, try to think of some of the places in your life, where you always got high, or in which you used to associate with getting high, then "turn over" one of them! "Turn over" one place today and see how it feels.

October 15

Being of Service

"We are spiritually aware. We become of service—at home, on the job, and in our fellowship of recovery."

- Life with Hope, second edition, page 67

The power of working the Twelve Steps is revealed as I persevere in my recovery journey. I benefited from a thorough examination of my past, and found I can move forward unburdened from my past transgressions. I discovered that I can now lead a useful life. By developing a meaningful, ongoing relationship with a Higher Power, I learned the rewards of living by the spiritual principles my program has taught me.

Shifting my motivation away from fear and self-centeredness to the spiritually enriching values of honesty, willingness, humility, faith, courage, hope, acceptance, and forgiveness led to achieving a spiritual awakening. Being of service to my family, friends, colleagues, and fellows in recovery is a natural extension of this awakening.

It can be profoundly beneficial to be of service. Sometimes the service is easy for me; at other times it requires faith that God is taking care of me as I do things I considered unimaginable. I accept all as growth opportunities and recognize God's blessing to have them.

Final thought: Today, I will strive to be of service as it manifests my gratitude for the gifts I have received as a result of working my recovery program.

October 16

The God Hole

"Step Two: Came to believe that a power greater than ourselves could restore us to sanity."

- *Life with Hope*, first edition, page 5

Early in recovery I heard a number of stories about how we addicts try over and over to fill in for something missing in our lives. I felt empty. There's a hole in my heart; and I tried to fill that hole with pot, alcohol, food, sex, or any number of substances and activities. I came to understand both that the hole was unfathomable and that only a belief in a power greater than myself could relieve my cravings. It came to be known as the "God hole." My constant desire for love, identity, and self-satisfaction could be fulfilled in spiritual connection. "Coming to believe" is a process. I feel that this is illustrated in a story I read that says:

> I walk down the street and fall into a deep hole in the sidewalk. I feel lost and helpless but it isn't my fault. It takes me forever to find a way out.

> I walk down the same street and although I pretend not to see it, I fall into the same hole again. I can't believe I am in the same place but it isn't my fault. It still takes me a long time to get out.

> I walk down the same street and I see a deep hole in the sidewalk. I still fall in. It is a habit. This time my eyes are open and I know where I am. I get out immediately.

> I walk down the same street. There is a hole in the sidewalk but this time I walk around it.

> I walk down another street.

> Paraphrased from Autobiography in Five Chapters by Portia Nelson, 2012 edition

Final thought: Today, I'm guided by Higher Power on the road to recovery.

October 17

A Far Better Way of Life

"We do things that we could have never done alone."

- Life with Hope, third edition, page 45

My addiction to marijuana made me feel like my life had become shipwrecked. My life continued to spiral downward and became increasingly unmanageable. Smoking pot used to lift me up, but was now just dragging me down. I was no longer getting high; I was smoking to satisfy a craving that was out of control. I had become addicted and I was powerless. No amount of willpower set me free of my compulsion to smoke pot.

The Marijuana Anonymous program seemed to be heaven-sent. The Steps, the fellowship, reliance on a power greater than myself (aka God), and a willingness to practice the principles of the program have allowed me to now live a life that before recovery seemed unimaginable. The program has allowed me to "live of good purpose," be of service to others, and grow along spiritual lines. Seeking spiritual progress, rather than perfection, has been a blessing.

Final thought: I am grateful to be set free from my addiction and set on an ever-rewarding journey of spiritual growth and development.

October 18

Living Clean

"We were not problem users whose problems went away when we threw away our stash. When we stopped using, we found we had a problem with living; we were addicts."

- Life with Hope, second edition, page 6

This quote, to me, is the definition and core presentation of addiction. It is not the marijuana use itself, but my inability to live life exactly as it is, exactly the way I am: clean. When I quit smoking weed, I thought that everything would immediately be fixed. What I found is that all of the rawest, darkest, and most terrifying parts of myself came to light and my life felt more unmanageable than ever.

I couldn't understand why everyone in the meetings seemed so happy and spoke so highly of their lives without weed. I briefly pondered the conspiracy that everyone was lying about this "magic" of recovery. I kept coming back like they said. I found a sponsor. We worked the Steps together. One day, I realized that I was one of those people in meetings saying how much better my life was now that I was clean. Addiction is the deep internal obsession with the fixing, managing, and controlling of other people, places, things, and ideas. When I got caught up in this cycle, I tended to use substances to numb this lack of control.

When I surrender to life on life's terms, and live in the moments as they pass, fully, presently, and cleanly, I find relief from this obsession. Recovery has shown me that living clean is the best way to live, as it is the only way to live in which I am not yearning for anything other than exactly what I have.

Final thought: Today, I remember that living clean is the solution to my addict obsession to fix, manage, and control. I will live in the moments as they pass, one day at a time.

October 19

Honest with Myself

"We had to look honestly at our relationship with marijuana and its effect on our lives."

- *Life with Hope*, second edition, page 1

I always knew I had a problem with marijuana and that it was detrimental to my life as far back as high school when I became a daily user. I was unwilling to change or give up smoking despite my family's pleas over the years and even an ultimatum from my partner later in life. Sitting alone in my parent's living room after a divorce, wondering how I got there, I was able to see the real impact my choices had on my life and the ones I loved. I realized I had chosen marijuana over so many things, including my partner and my marriage. I could be honest with myself and others and accept that it was a problem worth doing something about.

Final thought: When I was able to be honest about my marijuana use and the damage it caused in my life, I was able to move forward and begin the process of recovery.

October 20

For Fun and For Free

"We are simply addicts of equal status, freely helping each other."

- Life with Hope, second edition, page 89

I first attended an MA meeting at the urging of my therapist, and after a few years clean, I decided to enter the mental health field myself. Therapy was a lifesaver for me—it both got me into, and enhanced, my recovery—and I was excited to share that lifesaving gift with others!

Once I entered the field, Tradition Eight took on a new meaning for me. I was taught by my sponsor and others that my 12-Step work with newcomers should always be for fun and for free (a.k.a. "nonprofessional"), while at work I learned that not every client with a marijuana problem needs or wants a 12-Step answer.

Now, Tradition Eight helps me remember that when I attend a meeting, I get to be just one recovering member among many. My recovery experiences can help me have empathy for my clients, but at MA, I get to take off my therapist "hat" and focus on just taking care of me. What a relief!

Final thought: What "hat" am I wearing when I attend a meeting? Am I trying to play the expert, or a member among members?

October 21

What is Recovery?

"We are all unique examples of how the program works, each of us with our distinct gifts to share."

- Life with Hope, second edition, page 69

I made this list when asked, "how do you define recovery?"

A willingness to continue to go to meetings,

A willingness to continue to work the Steps,

Not being unconsciously bound to old patterns,

Not reacting in old ways,

Giving myself time and permission to feel my feelings,

Making choices based on the present,

Being able to take chances and to risk,

Being open and vulnerable with other people,

Allowing myself to be happy, joyous and free,

Being one in a community with other addicts,

Reaching out to my sponsor or a friend when needed,

Being willing to have a sponsor and be a sponsor,

Using the tools of daily prayer and meditation,

Never feeling alone anymore,

Knowing I have a Higher Power, even if I can't define it, and

Using all the recovery tools in my spiritual toolkit.

Final thought: Today and every day, my recovery is the priority of my life; without it, I may not have a life.

October 22

Powerless Every Day

"We learned that we could not control our using."

- Life with Hope, second edition, page 1

I was completely bewildered when I entered recovery and people kept saying that their Higher Power was keeping them clean and sober. This didn't make any sense to me. If my Higher Power wanted me to be clean and sober, why did I use for so long, and why was it so hard to quit? When I was told I had no control or power over marijuana and other drugs, I rebelled. Didn't I come into recovery? I was making decisions to come to meetings and work the steps with a sponsor. What did my Higher Power have to do with it?

Slowly, over time, the fog lifted and I realized that I truly am powerless over marijuana, and when I forget that I am powerless, my life is unmanageable. I need to remind myself about Step One every day. Then I turn my will and my life (my thoughts and my actions) over to a higher power, whether I understand it or not.

Final thought: Today, I ask to be reminded that I am always powerless over marijuana, and my life is unmanageable if I forget.

October 23

One Addict Helping Another

"The therapeutic value of one addict helping another is without parallel, because only another addict can identify with and offer recovery to a newcomer by sharing experience, strength, and hope."

- *Life with Hope*, second edition, page 81

MA's primary purpose is to carry the message of recovery to the still suffering addict. We do this in meetings, and through sponsorship. It was a huge relief to me when I entered recovery to find other addicts who understood how treacherous this disease of addiction had been, and how hard it was to quit. I had tried to do it on my own, and was unable. I quickly learned that if I kept going to meetings, I would learn what I needed to stay clean. By listening to other addicts share their experience, strength, and hope, I could identify and start to use the tools they used.

I remember hearing people suggest that it was a good idea to stay in the center; to come to the meeting early, and stay after, and to sit in the midst of the group. It would've been easy to come late, and sit at the back, so I could go unnoticed, but I've found that newcomers are always welcomed. It took some months to be able to share a difficulty while going through it. I didn't know how to be vulnerable, so I didn't share a problem until it was solved. Eventually, I knew it would serve me better to share all of me, not just what I thought was acceptable. When I share all of me, the newcomer has a chance to identify and see themselves in whatever it is I'm dealing with. By sharing my experience, strength, and hope, the newcomer learns the tools to use to live a life in recovery.

Final thought: Today, I share my experience, strength, and hope with other addicts in recovery.

297

October 24

A Life Worth Living

"What a reward this program has given me—my life back!"

- I Needed It to Feel OK, *Life with Hope*, second edition, page 156

Before recovery, from the time I became addicted to marijuana, I didn't live my life. I started smoking pot when I was 15, and had become a full-blown addict by the time I was 19, consuming pot every waking minute. My main purpose in life was to get and use marijuana. I was merely existing, where each day was the same as the day before. Of course, I didn't realize that this was not how life was supposed to be lived while in the denial of my addiction.

I remember the first time I heard the Second Step about being restored to sanity. I wasn't sure I had ever been sane! Through working the program to the best of my ability, I have been given a life truly worth living. I am able to be of service to others. I am able to enjoy my day, and not just endure it. I have gratitude in my life and a deep appreciation of the beauty that exists all around me. I am connected to everyone and everything. These are gifts that have come to me by virtue of working the Twelve Steps of Marijuana Anonymous, and being part of this worldwide fellowship.

Final thought: Today, I am grateful that I have a life worth living.

October 25

Building Blocks of Growth

"We start to accept the unpleasantness in our lives and become grateful when we are able to experience growth from it."

- Life with Hope, second edition, page 68

Pain is often the price for our most important growth. Well before entering recovery, I learned to view my own personal struggles with depression and obsessive compulsive disorder as a means to have compassion for others who might have their own difficulties. Still, many days were filled with an inner strain to accept my imperfections, while trying to maintain faith that I could lead a successful and productive life despite them. Years of using pot to cope with (really, mostly ignore) my negative feelings did nothing to lift the despair of what I imagined a life without such troubles might have been like.

In recovery, I have found that feelings of grief and despair that come with experiences of loss or challenge can be building blocks to cultivating my relationship with my Higher Power. It requires an awareness and openness to the idea that difficult experiences are a gift. This leads me to reflect and pray about the lessons that help me move forward with my life. How can I experience growth from something unpleasant—or even terrible? After some time, I am often surprised to find that I can be grateful for what my Higher Power has helped me learn.

Final thought: Today, I accept that God directs my personal growth in ways that, while not always obvious or necessarily pleasant, assists me in becoming a better human being.

October 26

Why Marijuana Anonymous?

"We strive for progress, not perfection."

- *Life with Hope*, first edition, page 33

I have been in recovery for a long time. Newcomers to our MA meetings ask, "Why do I feel I need Marijuana Anonymous? Am I afraid I'll go out? Do I have cravings? Am I only here to carry the message?" Other 12-Step meetings also have helped me stay clean all of these years.

Before I came to MA, I worked the Steps, had a sponsor, stayed clean and sober, but I had to keep quiet about my pot; my favorite, my precious. When I got high for the first time; it was like finding God. I remember every moment from the second I realized I was stoned until I stumbled into bed four hours later. I was a teenage alcoholic, but marijuana saved me from alcoholism. My friends, my lovers, my lifestyle, where I lived, what I ate, and what kind of parent I became, were affected by pot. Now that I attend MA meetings, I can talk about these things and I can work the Steps from my real self.

Final thought: Today, I understand that marijuana addiction is a disease. Only with the help of my Higher Power, sponsorship, working with others, working the Steps, will I progress in recovery.

October 27

Working the Steps

"We were not problem users whose problems went away when we threw away our stash. When we stopped using, we found we had a problem with living; we were addicts."

- *Life with Hope*, first edition, page 6

Marijuana is just a symptom of the real problem, me. My thoughts and actions are just not right. I have both a feeling of grandiosity and low self-esteem. I think I'm not good enough, and that no one loves or likes me. I used marijuana to cope with these feelings. Now that I'm not using, I really feel those feelings. There is a solution, the Twelve Steps.

When I work the Steps, I begin to recover. These feelings do not have power over me anymore. I get some peace and serenity. Through the Steps I am able to clear up the wreckage of the past, repair my relationships with others, and connect with a Higher Power of my own understanding.

I can live my life again. I get to be a productive worker at my job. I am reliable for my family and friends. I am a useful member of society. One day at a time, I don't use. With the Steps in my life, I recover.

Final thought: Today, I will work the Steps and recover.

October 28

Is My Life Really Unmanageable?

"Step One: *We admitted we were powerless over marijuana, that our lives had become unmanageable.*"

- *Life with Hope*, first edition, page 1

I came into Marijuana Anonymous when I realized I could not control or stop using marijuana; however, Step One asked me to say my life was unmanageable. I was functioning, had a good job, was supporting myself; I was even being an active parent and community member. When I looked up the word unmanageable I found it means "difficult or impossible to control or manage." This allowed me to identify and say Step One honestly and start my journey in MA.

Final thought: Today, regardless if I am at day one or day 5000, reflecting on how my life is unmanageable, I know that a Higher Power of my understanding will help me do what I cannot do alone.

October 29

Living the Solution

"Our program is not easy, but it is simple."

- How It Works, *Life with Hope*, first edition, page 103

I was talking with someone who has long-time recovery. We were discussing the fundamentals of recovery. I was told that there are three suggested acronyms for keeping recovery. Remembering these acronyms helps to keep it simple.

The first is ODAAT; One Day at a Time. I can succeed in my recovery if I concentrate on today, not yesterday, not tomorrow. I am clean and sober today. It can be overwhelming to think that I need to be clean and sober for the rest of my life; I just have to think about today. If I remember this every day, it will get easier along the way.

Next is HOW, which refers to Honest, Open, and Willing; the first three Steps of recovery. I know that I have to be Honest about being an addict. If I stay in denial I won't face reality and I won't begin to change. I need to be Open to asking for help; I can't do this alone. I rely on the wisdom shared by other addicts in recovery. I am Willing to let go of self-control. I can't find recovery by relying on self-will; I need to have faith and trust others.

Last is NOW; No Other Way. I try to remember that there is No Other Way to recovery. Having a spiritual connection helps me with my recovery. I don't need to do this alone; I can ask for help. Remembering all of these things helps me to live in the solution.

Final thought: Today, I will remember that recovery is simple if I just remember to live in the solution.

October 30

Take What You Need and Leave the Rest

"...principles before personalities..."

- *Life with Hope,* first edition, page 99

While using, I did not care if it was a person I hated or not, if they could get me high then I was spending time with them. Once I got clean, I decided that I would do the exact opposite of what I did before. I decided if I did not like a person I wouldn't go near them or listen to them. I found myself at a meeting where someone said something completely off the wall and I remember thinking, "Wow, how can I relate to a person like that?" I started to wonder if I belonged at all; a few told me, "Take what you need and leave the rest."

At the next meeting, that same person said something that I truly needed to hear that day and I realized that we do not have to relate to everything about one another to learn from each other. Sometimes, a person may offend you one day and say exactly what you need to hear the next day.

Final thought: Today, I will learn to put "principles before personalities" in my recovery.

October 31

Unity

"The concept of unity, and all that it stands for, helps preserve the fellowship."

- *Life with Hope*, second edition, page 73

Unity is a concept that is so crucial to our program that it is the cornerstone of the first Tradition. As a newcomer, this idea was lost on me. I was only thinking of myself and how I was being served by the program. This was an important place to be at the time because I was learning a different way to live life. However, as I kept coming back I began to see this idea with new eyes.

I want to show up on time to the meeting so that my entrance doesn't pull focus away from the person speaking as I'm trying to find my seat. This idea was not something I ever thought of before sobriety. Learning this concept in the program has led me to use it in other areas of my life. When I practice this concept in my work environment it contributes to my ability to be a team player. I recently had a conflict with a co-worker. She and I wanted to do something differently. I applied this Tradition and asked myself, "What is our common ground here?" We each wanted to help our clients. Breaking the concept of unity down to a simple question helped me to look at my conflict with new eyes. This led me to think of how to combine our two differing ideas in order to serve our community. Unity is something that holds us together, whether at work or in meetings.

Final thought: Today, I will keep in mind how to contribute to the unity of my group.

November 1

The Miracle

"In recovery, we begin to develop a relationship with a Higher Power, or renew one that we once had. We come to believe in a God of our own individual understanding, a Higher Power that will help us in all phases of our lives. Some of us believed that dependence meant restrictiveness. However, many of us have found that dependence on a Higher Power means freedom of choice and freedom to grow as individuals."

- Life with Hope, first edition, page 56

It took me several years to get off pot, but that came as no surprise as I had spent over half my life using it as much as possible. Once I found the right sponsor, I was given a simple program to follow, and I decided to follow those suggestions like my life depended on it. I was sick and tired of spending a few months smoking and then trying to quit again.

Working with my sponsor, I was finally able to develop an honest relationship, and he in turn helped me develop a relationship with my Higher Power. Staying honest also meant acknowledging that I still wished I could smoke pot. Anytime the desire came up, I would fast-forward the movie in my head and it was enough to keep me from taking that first puff. After 50 months off weed, I realized that the miracle had finally happened to me too. I was healing from a surgery when I realized that I had made it through some of the scariest moments of my life without weed.

As I used to smoke to deal with my fears, I have now learned that the Serenity Prayer and this fellowship are more powerful than any joint. The desire to smoke weed had finally been lifted. I was finally granted a new sense of freedom. All I had to do was not smoke today, and come back tomorrow.

Final thought: Today, I am grateful that I no longer need weed to deal with my fears. Today, I have new tools and new friends.

November 2

Embrace the Mystery

"For many of us, our addiction to marijuana came as we sought a greater reality, or even a mystical experience through the drug."

- Life with Hope, first edition, page 55

When I used marijuana, I thought I was gaining clarity and getting closer to my Higher Power. Instead, I became socially isolated and withdrawn. Weed became my Higher Power. Self-centeredness was my form of devotion. I know all too well where the use of marijuana will lead. It isn't a very long path, and there isn't much to see at the end of it. I have already spent far too much time here. There is no mystery left for me in the return to addiction.

The path of sobriety, on the other hand, remains a complete mystery. Every day, I wake up with wonder at what will happen today. I do not know where this path of recovery leads and my curiosity will keep me sober for today.

I have seen the program work miracles in those around me who work the program. I was told early on to stick with those actively working the program, and that allowed me to become humble enough to ask a fellow addict to become my sponsor. This led to self-discovery through the 12 Steps. I have become a kind person again. The journey of recovery is filled with excitement and wonder. With each prayer or meditation, I move further along this mysterious path. As I seek conscious contact with my Higher Power, I remember I am no longer in this alone. The road to addiction is all too familiar. It does not lead to where I want to go. The program takes me where I failed to go through marijuana use.

Final thought: Today, I will revel at the mystery of life and be grateful for the opportunity to walk a path that leads somewhere I have not yet been.

November 3

Spiritual Principles

"We use these spiritual principles to guide our behavior."

- *Life with Hope*, third edition, page 60

The spiritual principles have become a guide for giving me direction. Principles such as honesty, humility, open mindedness, patience, tolerance, faith, and integrity are some that I have tried to follow. Even now that I am clean, my life becomes unmanageable if I am not living in line with the principles. I can take a situation or a reaction I am having and line it up against the principles to check in with what is the next right thing to do.

Time and time again, my perspective grows as I use all the principles in harmony. They are interlinked, interwoven and become more meaningful when used in combination; that is where I grow. It alleviates justifications, excuses, and linear thinking as I run through the principles. If I am in judgment, I am not practicing the principle of open-mindedness, nor am I practicing humility if I think I know everything enough to cast judgment. I am not practicing justice because to sit in judgment is not fair. When I feel so strongly that I am right, that I need to convince others or voice my opinion, the more I need to stop. Can I trust my Higher Power, and accept that I am not anyone else's Higher Power?

Acting with integrity takes courage, because sometimes doing the right thing is not easy. Knowing what is the right thing to do takes reflection, willingness, openness to different perspectives and different options. When I persevere I will figure out the right thing to do. These spiritual principles are interlinked, not to be used solo.

Final thought: Just for today, I will practice all these principles and practice applying them together to align myself with my Higher Power and with what is best for my spiritual growth.

November 4

Let Go and Let God

"We come to learn that our 'first instincts' are often bad indicators of the proper path. We find that if we put top priority on spiritual growth, it is less likely that self-will and character defects will pull us down."

- Life with Hope, first edition, page 60

Many of us in recovery have heard about "The Committee." It's the constant stream of voices running in my head, giving me advice and/or a hard time. I prefer, though, to think in terms of thought-gears running in my head. The little ones almost never stop turning, but it's the big ones that'll get me.

I think "First Gear" is that constant stream of thoughts and stories running in my head. "Second Gear" is when these thoughts become loud, and I start to give attention to them. "Third Gear" is when I start to truly believe them, and even my body reacts to them with fear, anxiety or anger. "Fourth Gear" is when they've taken over my actions and feelings completely—I don't even notice them anymore. "Fifth Gear" is pretty much full freakout mode or relapse.

Stopping that First Gear is experiencing the calm, centered mind. It's pretty much the whole point of meditation. I think it's more practical and important to simply notice that First Gear is turning, and not let the Second Gear to get into gear. Noticing the First Gear and not engaging the Second Gear, while taking action, can also be called facing fears. When the Second Gear starts going, fear can cause paralysis. Sometimes, First Gear can be an indicator that I have something deeper to work on. I can engage with it as a helper, turning on the light inside, looking around in the dark corners, and seeing what's in there. If I can get this down, maybe I can even be grateful for the "problem" of my little thought-gears.

Final thought: Today, I am going to stop my thought-gears from gaining control in my head and remember to "let go and let God."

November 5

Spiritual Connection

"We find that if we put top priority on spiritual growth, it is less likely that self-will and character defects will pull us down."

- Life with Hope, first edition, page 60

Through working the Steps of Marijuana Anonymous with my sponsor and doing my best to practice the spiritual principles of the program, I've developed a relationship with my Higher Power that I never imagined was possible. For me, spiritual growth comes through the actions I take to work my program: working the Steps, calling my sponsor, fellowship, service, daily prayer and meditation, and reading the literature. I express gratitude to my Higher Power every day for recovery and for the blessings in my life, even when I don't always feel grateful.

Every morning, I start my day by making conscious contact with God, and asking for guidance to do the next right thing. Sometimes, my ego can get in the way, but I've learned to apply faith and self-forgiveness to all situations and problems. Each time I take an action using the spiritual tools of the program, my recovery grows stronger and I'm less likely to default to my self-will. I am more likely to act towards myself and others with kindness, love, and understanding.

Marijuana Anonymous has not only given me freedom from marijuana, but also peace, serenity, and an ability to be of service to my fellow humans. What a miracle!

Final thought: Today, I am will prioritize my recovery by making time for prayer and meditation.

November 6

Building a Relationship

"In recovery, we begin to develop a relationship with a Higher Power, or renew one that we once had."

- Life with Hope, first edition, page 56

I walked into the rooms of Marijuana Anonymous alienated by the faith with which I was raised. Additionally, many newcomers are completely turned off by the references in our literature and from shares in meetings about God and Higher Power. This makes perfect sense in the context of being an addict with no experience or understanding of the program of Marijuana Anonymous. As an addict, the last thing that I personally wanted was someone telling me what to do, and I certainly didn't want anyone telling me who and what to believe in.

Fortunately, those who keep coming back find out that they can believe in anything they want to, as long as it is a power greater than themselves. This is where the suggestions end. The relationship one has with a Higher Power is one of the most personal and fulfilling relationships one can cultivate in recovery. It needs no justification, no description, no explanation, no road map, and no discussion. It belongs to you, and if it works for you, God bless you.

Final thought: Today, I am open to building a relationship with a power greater than myself.

311

November 7

Working the Steps Brings Hope

"Our message is a simple one of hope: by following the spiritual principles of the Twelve Steps, any addict can stop using marijuana and lose the obsession and desire to do so."

- Life with Hope, third edition, page 58

Most of the years of my life were run by obsession with marijuana and constant desire to use it; that was my way of life. My hopes centered around that on a daily basis. Living any other way had never even occurred to me. Eventually, I reached the point where I was desperately addicted. I was faced with the undeniable need to change; I felt completely hopeless. Attending meetings, getting a sponsor, and working the Steps soon taught me I am powerless.

My deepest hope is for a program of recovery which would lead me to a power greater than myself, greater than marijuana, and the disease of addiction. Working the Twelve Steps brings hope and the spiritual principles to life. Following the spiritual principles gives a kind of hope that I'd never known before recovery. Now, working my program each day, the old obsession and desire to use is gone and has been replaced with the hope of this better life in recovery.

Final thought: We remember, that as long as there is life, there is hope. Our hope depends on a Higher Power; that hope and power come to life in working the Twelve Steps.

November 8

Faith in God's Will

"Faith provides us with the motivation to surrender to God's will."

- Life with Hope, second edition, page 57

As an active addict, I was a very negative person. I was enslaved by marijuana, and one day I was led to the rooms of recovery, where I have learned a new way to live, free from addiction. I learned how to pray in Marijuana Anonymous. At first, I would recite the prayers I heard in the meetings: the Third and Seventh Step Prayers and the Serenity Prayer. I heard that I should not ask for my will, but ask to be shown my Higher Power's will. This wasn't easy for me, because I could not always tell what was my will versus what was my Higher Power's will. I've come to understand that my intuition is one of my Higher Power's voices, and if I listen to it, it gets louder.

The Eleventh Step reminds me to pray for my Higher Power's will for me and for the power to carry that out. I didn't like the saying, "your will, not mine," so I changed it to, "may my will, be your will." In recovery, I want to keep my life as positive as I can.

Final thought: Higher Power, show me your will for me today, and grant me the power to carry it out. May my will, be your will.

November 9

Powerlessness Leads to Choice

"...surrender outweighs the illusion of control and becomes our only option for recovery."

- Life with Hope, second edition, page 3

When I first got clean, I knew I was powerless over marijuana, but I didn't think my life was unmanageable. I had a job, an apartment, a cat, and a partner. Slowly, as the cloud of smoke left my brain, I realized that using pot every minute I was awake, even though I was no longer getting high, made my life completely unmanageable. My thinking and the constant craving for pot was unmanageable.

Once I realized that the entire First Step was relevant to my life, I could surrender to my powerlessness and unmanageability. Each surrender to the Steps has been a huge gift. Working these Twelve Steps has been the only thing that has made real and lasting change in my life. I have a set of tools which help me live happy, joyous, and free, in a way I could never have imagined before recovery.

Final thought: Today, I am grateful for another day clean, and pray to stay that way.

November 10

Step Eleven

"When we regularly seek...expansion through prayer and meditation, rather than marijuana use, we find that we are increasingly fulfilled..."

- Life with Hope, first edition, page 55

If my perception is inherently limited, if I am stuck with my own subjectivity, then how am I supposed to not only accept that we are all interconnected, let alone experience that elusive unity? For me, this is my mission, given to me as the greatest gift of the 12 Steps of Marijuana Anonymous. I get to seek, through prayer and meditation, to improve my conscious contact with, and awareness of, this unity. My prayers and meditations are not designed to get anything other than to remember the unity. I need to remind myself of this each and every moment, that's just how it has to be.

Final thought: Today, when I remember that we are all a part of, that being together is the only way, then I am ready to be the best I can be, an integral part of the whole, receptive to the unity.

November 11

Finding Joy

"With gratitude, we can share our happiness and increase our sense of joy, peace, and security."

- Life with Hope, first edition, pages 58-59

Happiness is:

A sunny field of daffodils,

Seeing a rainbow after a storm,

Sunshine on a spring day,

Watching your baby take its first steps,

Sitting by the fire on a cold day,

Looking at a blue sky and breathing the fresh air,

Seeing the beautiful colors in nature,

Hearing the birds sing in your garden,

Listening to the surf at the ocean,

Hearing a waterfall,

Appreciating the stormy days knowing there will be better days ahead,

Knowing that you have done the best you can,

Being able to forgive yourself and others,

Feeling at peace with yourself,

Loving yourself,

Offering help to someone in need,

Receiving a smile from a friend,

Having no expectations of a friend,

Having friends who love you and

People in your life who help create wonderful memories.

Final thought: Every day, I thank my Higher Power for another day in recovery so that I can experience this happiness and joy, instead of the sadness of addiction.

November 12

A Loving Presence

"Through prayer and meditation, we are brought over and over again into contact with a loving Presence. We sense the healing force of God in our lives."

- Life with Hope, second edition, page 60

My prayer:

"Divine Presence, which is in all of life, help me today to remember that you are always here. I am never alone, and your guidance is always available. How do I access your support? All I need to do is ask. Ask for an intuitive thought, or guidance, or comfort, and it will come in its own time. Being human, I don't always remember to ask or to wait for an answer to my prayers. As an addict, I want what I want when I want it. I am grateful to be learning a new way of moving through the world with your help. Please channel your love and guidance through me so that I may be an instrument of your love, grace, and abundance. Help me remember that I am held in your loving embrace at all times. You know us better than we know ourselves. Humor us, as we trudge along the road of happy destiny."

Final thought: Today, I seek the guidance of my Higher Power in all I do.

November 13

Attitude of Gratitude

"The practice of gratitude is perhaps the most moving and powerful way in which we can cultivate a conscious contact with a Higher Power."

- Life with Hope, first edition, page 58

Conscious awareness of the many things for which I am grateful strengthens my sense of connection—the source that keeps me clean and sober. This is God as I understand God. God uses people to help me stay clean and sober. God can use me to help others; I cannot be much use to my fellows when I lack gratitude.

Life is easier when I focus on where I do have power. I have power over my attitude, and an attitude of gratitude is the way to go. Using the letters of the alphabet can help me think of things for which I am grateful. My awareness shifts to my Creator and all the blessings that are there for me to count, even in the midst of affliction.

Final thought: Today, I will share at least one thing that I am grateful for with someone.

November 14

Presence

"We came to believe in a loving, compassionate Presence..."

- Life with Hope, first edition, page 56

The process of coming to believe in a power greater than myself was not easy for me in the beginning of my recovery. I had spent a lifetime of disappointment in formal religion. I thought of myself as an agnostic and the closest I came to a spiritual connection was in nature. I also used my disbelief as an excuse for continuing to use.

In early recovery, along with going to meetings and working the Steps, I still had trouble with identifying with a Higher Power. As I meditated, I began to coordinate the phrase "let God, and let go" to my breath, so that with each inhalation, I would take in what I needed, and let go of what was wrong for me as I exhaled. I breathed in acceptance, and let go of control. I breathed in courage, and let go of fear. As I continued, I found myself saying, "Let me be present, and let go of the future. Let presence be, and let go of the past." This was the moment when it dawned on me that presence was my Higher Power.

I came to the realization that as long as I remained present, I felt connected to something larger than myself. I didn't have to do this alone. Meditation is one of the gifts of recovery. The practice of emptying my mind, focusing my breath, and staying present has provided the serenity promised in Marijuana Anonymous.

Final thought: Feeling God as a presence in my life means I don't have to do this alone.

November 15

Mindfulness Practice

"As we let loose our grip on the reins of our lives, we find we are being led, slowly and certainly, in the right direction—towards home."

- *Life with Hope*, first edition, page 57

Being mindful is the foundation for my meditation. When I'm in the present, I can trust in the presence of a power greater than myself. There is a connection to "this power" that I strive to improve when I can, and I try all the time. Working to improve this connection is like expanding the space in my mindfulness to sustain a kind of "God's presence," ideally, all throughout the day. Seeing my thoughts and feelings as they arise gives me a chance to effectively let go of them before they become triggering. This foundation eliminates a lot of my problems.

Mindfulness practice in turn has many benefits for me. It allows me to be aware of what's happening in the moment and allows my Higher Power to help me as I need it. This path, which is ever-changing, is my focus in recovery. Practice mindfulness then distractions and illusions will lessen. Love, patience, peace of mind, compassion, happiness and understanding of the true nature of things will be cultivated.

By seeing through "perfect awareness," I intuitively know what I have to do in the moment. It is kind of a "spiritual guide." When I make this connection and experience it working in my life, making a difference to me in tangible ways, my ability to maintain conscious contact grows stronger. My faith in that connection to a power greater than myself grows stronger. This practice is bearing fruit in my recovery and adds joy to my life as I build healthy relationships and spiritually-based connections.

Final thought: Today, I will practice mindfulness and my recovery will grow.

November 16

The Blank Canvas

"Many of us have trouble distinguishing between God's will and self-will."

- *Life with Hope*, third edition, page 53

I know that I often struggle with this, distinguishing between what is my Higher Power's will and what is my own. Many times a thousand thoughts are rushing through my mind: what I need from the grocery store; how I don't like what someone at work said; frustrations and joys from the relationships in my life; and more. These thoughts are my subconscious mind's attempt at imposing its will on my life through my thoughts. I am not my thoughts. I am the space between them which holds those thoughts tightly, until they are dealt with in a way that lets them float away into space, away from the front of my mind, either to be forgotten, or to be tucked away somewhere as a memory I might recall later in life. I am not my thoughts or feelings, just as the chalkboard is not the chalk, and the canvas is not the paint.

I have thoughts and feelings, but I am far more than just those thoughts and feelings. The next time I meditate, as I become aware of those scribbles of chalk on my chalkboard mind, I acknowledge them, and try to let them go. I might immediately notice another thought scribbled on my mind, but I let that one go too. The thoughts will still be there later. It may take much practice to simply be the blank slate of the chalkboard, separated from the chalk, but if I am able to connect with the feeling of being the blank canvas, then I too may find better clarity on what is my Higher Power's will, and what is my own self-will.

Final thought: Today, I will be the canvas, and I will let my Higher Power be the painter.

November 17

The Twelve Principles

"Our best thinking brought us to our bottom."

- *Life with Hope*, first edition, page 8

I love the saying, "Our best thinking brought us to our bottom." When I try to manipulate others and situations to get my way, I am again resorting to my own worst thinking. I figure if I can steer the bus in just the right way, I will get what I want and be happy and relieved of suffering. However, when my actions are based on self-will and ego gratification, even when I initially achieve what I want, the outcomes are often hollow and may have negative unintended consequences that become clear over time. My desires alone, and the means I use to get those desires fulfilled, if not aligned with the will of my Higher Power, can lead to suffering for myself and others.

The beautiful thing about recovery is that it provides me with basic principles that, much like a map, when followed leads to elegant, robust and long-lasting positive outcomes. When I make the principles of recovery my focus and act upon those, I no longer have to suffer from obstacles generated by my own worst thinking.

The principles of Honesty, Hope, Faith, Courage, Integrity, Willingness, Humility, Love, Discipline, Perseverance, Spiritual Awareness, and Service as learned and practiced through the Twelve Steps are the keys. With these keys, I align myself with the help and support of a power greater than myself. When I am troubled and don't know what to do, I pause, take a breath, and check-in to see if I am being willful or trying to manipulate people and situations; then I smile and turn the situation over to my Higher Power.

Final thought: Today, I ask God to reveal to me which recovery principle I need to focus on to get back to serenity.

November 18

MA is a "We" Program

"...practically everyone can easily and naturally draw strength and support from the fellowship."

- *Life with Hope*, first edition, page 7

When I started working the Steps, I learned how every single word of each Step has profound significance. My sponsor told me, "The first word of the First Step is 'we' for a reason. This is a 'we' program, not a 'me' program." This same sponsor suggested I call at least three members from the program every single day. Often when I reach out to help another, I benefit just as much, if not more. As I persist in regularly calling other members, I learn the power of this connection when I am struggling.

Likewise, through regular meeting attendance, I learn that I am not in this alone. Pain is inevitable in the program, but suffering is not. When I become upset or angry with other members, I remember that I am in the rooms because of a spiritual malady that requires helping each other. Together, we recover.

Final thought: Today, I will take time to connect with other members of the program, whether I am struggling or not.

November 19

The Spirit of Service

"Tradition Nine defines true fellowship: a group without organization, guided by a loving God, and driven only by the spirit of service."

- Life with Hope, second edition, page 92

When I first came into MA, I didn't understand how an organization could function without a leader. The Twelve Traditions seemed boring and irrelevant to help me stay clean and sober another day. Over time, I've learned that the Traditions help the group in a way similar to how the Steps help the individual. The Traditions give MA structure so that we can focus on our primary purpose of carrying the message to the marijuana addict who still suffers.

Given that I am an addict learning how to live a clean life, among other addicts, our groups can turn to the Traditions to keep us focused on the positive. MA works because we're not all sick on the same day. It works because we are all striving to live spiritual lives.

I heard early on that to keep my recovery I needed to give it away. This is the spirit of service. MA works because we welcome the newcomer, and offer the kind of support we received when we came in the rooms. When I share my recovery with a newcomer, I'm reminded of how much I've learned since my first day in recovery.

Even if I don't understand a concept of a Higher Power that governs our group conscience, I've seen it work over and over again. MA works because we step in to be of service to each other and the group. I love the reminder that no one person is in charge.

Final thought: Today, I will trust that MA is guided by a loving Higher Power, and that we all step up to be of service to each other to keep it working for the still suffering addict.

November 20

The Right Direction

"Faith provides us with the motivation to surrender to God's will. We are, in truth, under the care of God. As we let loose our grip on the reins of our lives, we find we are being led, slowly and certainly, in the right direction—towards home."

- *Life with Hope*, first edition, page 57

The longer I am sober, the stronger my faith becomes and I see God's will in my life with clarity. When I am struggling with any question, at that moment, I do not have to make any decision. Making a decision, at all, is not God's will. When I let go of the need to do, to act, or to decide, and instead wait, God clearly (and often with a sense of humor) shows me the right decision path. When I rush to make a decision in my time, I am taking my will back. When I trust that the right path will open up for me, I am always clearly shown what to do. God speaks to me through "coincidences" and shows me what needs to be done. As long as I am actively listening and not doing, I will see God's path for me and it is better than what I would have "figured out" for myself.

Final thought: I will pause if I am unsure and wait for God to direct me.

November 21

Sober Vacations

"I always had a life. Thanks to Marijuana Anonymous, I now have a life worth living."

- A Life Worth Living, *Life with Hope*, third edition, page 143

When I was using marijuana, vacations were basically smoke-a-thons. I chose vacation destinations that would make scoring and using marijuana as easy as possible and I spent as much time as possible smoking, which was even more than what I usually smoked! This caused me to miss out on a lot of fun because of the need to be hidden away smoking, and then the lack of energy that came from using so much.

When I got clean, I was actually afraid of vacations. Would I ever be able to stay clean on a vacation? Would I even be able to enjoy the vacation? What would happen when I returned home? Thanks to Marijuana Anonymous, today I can use the tools of the program to plan and enjoy clean vacations. I can take an inventory on how I approached vacations in the past and learn what my part was in making past vacations smoke-a-thons. Since the marijuana fog has lifted from my brain, I can choose destinations and travel partners wisely.

Because I don't stay clean by myself, I can ask my Higher Power, my sponsor, and friends in the fellowship for wisdom and support. I can even attend MA meetings while I am on vacation, whether in-person, on the phone, or online. When I return home, I can check in with my MA support network to help with any "post-vacation blues," then I can gratefully share my experience, strength, and hope with others who want to plan and enjoy a sober vacation.

Final thought: Today, I will use the tools of the program to imagine, plan, and/or enjoy a sober vacation.

November 22

Hope to Grow

"We have received a gift that, in fact, amounts to a new state of being. We realize that our potential is limitless. We now have the tools to help us grow."

- Life with Hope, first edition, page 63

I thought I had a beautiful garden. It was amazing how I did nothing and the weeds grew to create greens, yellows, purples, oranges, and browns. I loved all the natural colors, but was powerless over their spread. A fellow lover of gardens, my neighbor, invited me over to show me hers. It was something I could have never imagined. There were beautiful flowers, bushes, trees, and plants.

I wanted what she had and saw how narrow my vision had become. I did not know where to start. She showed me where to go to get help. I met others there who loved the beauty of the natural world. I met fellows who could show me how to grow my garden. I explored different types of flowers and plants, was shown how they flourish, and introduced soils for their foundations.

I began to show up here every week to accept all the experience I could to grow my garden. I found tools here, steps to bringing life into my garden, and support and guidance when my plants would not thrive. My garden is beautiful today. It's not always what I want, but exactly what I need. Some plants don't do well in my garden while others love the light in my yard. I have to remember to work at my recovery every day and water my garden.

Now with strength and experience of my own, I can share this with others and spread hope that they too can have hope to grow a garden of their own. This is my recovery.

Final thought: Today, I remember I need meetings, sober fellows, a sponsor, the Steps, slogans, and literature to grow.

November 23

Higher Power's Guidance

"For each step we take towards God, God takes a thousand steps towards us."

- Life with Hope, first edition, page 56

The Eleventh Step is about communication with our Higher Power, something we can do every day. We have heard it said in 12-Step meetings that while praying is talking to our Higher Power, during meditation we make the stillness that allows our Higher Power to guide and talk to us.

I stopped these practices when I started smoking. I never started in the first place; either way it is never too late to learn and begin again. Prayer is about thanking as well as asking, and my Higher Power answers all my prayers; sometimes the answer isn't what I want it to be. Sometimes the answer to a plea is, "I'm sorry, but no," or "not yet," or "instead of that, how about this?" When I thank my Higher Power in prayer, I always receive a "you're welcome" in return.

If I am aware of the world around me; the people, the situations in which I find myself, or moments in nature, I might find the answers to my prayers there. Meditation enhances and hones my awareness. It separates the mud of my inner self into earth, air and water, making one thing distinguishable from another. Sometimes meditation answers prayers I wasn't even conscious of—like a gentle suggestion I hadn't yet considered, or a feeling of oneness with the universe that I hadn't experienced, a sense of belonging, or a taste of serenity.

Final thought: Today, I will ask my Higher Power to keep me sober today, and before going to sleep tonight, I will thank my Higher Power for having kept me sober this day. In between, I will let my Higher Power speak to me.

November 24

Control

"I have had enough lessons to accept that control is an illusion. If I trust the inner guidance my Higher Power gives me then I will receive all I need and more."

- Coming Home, *Life with Hope*, second edition, page 215

Before surrendering to the program, I thought my life was over. Everything that I had worked so hard to control—my career, my relationships, my secret mental health struggles, my curated image of perfection and "having it all together"—had all been shattered overnight. On top of my own personal crises, the world was shutting down as a result of the Covid-19 pandemic, evoking uncertainty and powerlessness on a global level.

Strangely, though, with each passing day of being isolated in my apartment, attending MA meetings on Zoom, and fiercely praying for the ability to accept my Higher Power's will, I grew more peaceful than I had ever been in my entire life. I accepted the job loss, the broken relationships, the necessary relocation. Instead of trying to control my circumstances, I trusted them. I trusted that the adversity I was enduring was part of a master plan that my Higher Power has for my life—one that provides necessary lessons and opportunities for growth and spiritual maturity. The miracle happened when I realized that the harder I try to control my entire life, the more out of control my life gets.

Final thought: Today, peace comes from letting go and trusting the path my Higher Power has put me on.

November 25

Breathe

"Meditation can develop our coping skills and increase our serenity...
It does a better job of calming us down than any other substance we
can put in our bodies. It can reduce stress and promote peace of mind."

- Beginning Meditation: An Approach to Step 11, MA Pamphlet

When I was smoking, the only time I would take a deep, long breath
was when I'd get home from work and take the first hit off my pipe or
joint. The day's stress would leave me and my evening would begin, or
so I thought. When I finally stopped smoking, I did not know what to do
with my stress, then I remembered all the meditation and yoga classes I
had attended while high during my smoking years.

All the teachings which focused on the breath, breathing deeply and
to the back of my ribs were helpful. This, as well as attending meetings
with the literature and phone calls, helped to prevent me from totally
freaking out in my first few months. It made me deal with my stress.

It has now become such a part of me that I automatically breathe
deeply when I enter into stressful situations. One of the great gifts of my
recovery has been the ability to take long relaxing breaths and learning
how to soothe myself, something which I was not taught in my childhood
home or at school. Another positive effect from stopping smoking is that
my sense of smell has returned. I can walk around my neighborhood
and through the local parks and woods and smell the beautiful natural
smells of the roses and trees. This brings me back to nature and reminds
me of my Higher Power's creation. I now look to my Higher Power to
show me or remind me how to relax.

Final thought: Stop. Breathe in for a count of seven and out for a count of
eleven.

November 26

Action Through the Steps

"Once we made a decision to turn our will and our lives over to a Higher Power, it was imperative that we do just that. After all, the faith we acquired by taking Step Three meant very little if we did not follow it with immediate action."

- Life with Hope, second edition, page 15

Step Three is about a decision, but a decision means very little if I don't take action to carry it out. I may decide to make dinner; that doesn't mean dinner is made. I have to follow it with a series of actions: get groceries, prepare the ingredients, start the stove or oven, and cook the meal for dinner to actually get made. If I decide I want to get a degree, I don't suddenly have that education. I have to apply to schools, attend classes, write essays, and take exams in order to obtain that degree. A series of actions implements my decision.

My decision in Step Three means I take action to turn over my will and my life. I take action by working the rest of the Steps. I look at exactly what I am turning over by writing inventory in my Fourth Step, sharing that inventory with another in my Fifth Step, looking at my behaviors and character traits that I need to let go of in my Sixth and Seventh Steps, and making amends in Step Nine. Through a series of actions, the Steps, I carry out my decision. I continue to carry out that decision with daily reflection, prayer and meditation, being of service, and living by spiritual principles. These actions allow me to continually turn my thinking and actions over to a Higher Power.

Final thought: Today, I will take action through the Steps, tools of the program, and with spiritual principles to implement my decision and turn my will and life over to the care of my Higher Power.

November 27

Praying Only for God's Will

"The operative word in Step Eleven is 'only'. We need to keep in mind that we pray *only* for knowledge of God's will for us and the power to carry that out."

- Life with Hope, first edition, page 57

Too often and for years I have woken up, prostrated on the floor in front of the window with the sunrise peeping through, and prayed for my will to be met. Since I was praying every morning, I thought I was doing the Eleventh Step correctly. I would pray for the needs of my day; the desires of my want; the list of things that I need to get through my day which only God could help me with. This drove me toward more resentment when things didn't go as I had prayed for, or more aptly, requested.

As it's been said, the cause of suffering is desire. It was during a book study that the above line, and specifically one word, jumped out at me, and that word is "only"—Only makes me right-sized. I am not summoning a genie to grant me my daily wishes; I am only supposed to pray for my Higher Power's will for me and nothing more. What that is, is not up to me, and that is freeing, knowing that my Higher Power always has my best interest at heart.

The more understanding I have of God's will for me, the more fulfilling my life will be. Praying, for me, leads me to a laundry list of expectations that inevitably won't happen, knowing that expectations are resentments under construction.

Final thought: Praying only for God's will returns me to humility.

November 28

Beginning with Gratitude

"With gratitude, we can share our happiness and increase our sense of joy, peace, and security."

- *Life with Hope*, first edition, pages 58-59

I thank you for waking up clear-headed.

I thank you for the beauty and wonder that surrounds me.

I thank you for my home, and the people who love me.

I thank you for showing me to do Your will, and not mine.

I thank you for my daily blessings.

I thank you for my clarity and my health.

I thank you for lifting my desire to use.

I thank you for loving me no matter what, and for teaching me to love myself.

I thank you for showing me that gratitude is prayer, and that it creates true energy in my life.

Final thought: Today, I begin my day with gratitude. I thank you, my Higher Power, for the sun rising and for being alive.

November 29

Prayer and Meditation

"Prayer and meditation are a real source of power and strength in living our program."

- Life with Hope, first edition, page 56

I found it hard to sit with my thoughts before joining the fellowship. I did not see the point in prayer. My relationship with my Higher Power was nonexistent. I started off feeling uneasy in my body, but slowly came to terms with my emotions. No longer running from them, I am free to tune into my intuition. The endless grasping for more was reduced with every prayer, and now I feel calm as soon as I get on my knees.

The prayers started a dialogue with my Higher Power, and meditation gives me answers. With time to check-in, I am no longer trying to escape from myself. Now, I welcome the routine it gives me. Soon, I find that if I don't start the day with a prayer, I will feel off. Reaching out guides me to find answers in my life and I become a proactive player. No longer a passenger, I am learning to live fully in the here and now.

Final thought: Today, I will cherish prayer and meditation, and seek my Higher Power's influence.

November 30

Don't Leave Before the Miracle Happens

"Recovery does not happen all at once. It is a process, not an event."

- Life with Hope, first edition, page 4

I'm sitting here in awe of how I walked into these rooms with zero idea of the process that would unfold before me. My relationship to time was pretty unrealistic. I was always preoccupied with the past, regretting my missteps, and how my life had turned out. Also, I was afraid to move forward. It's why I would smoke—to make time stop, so I could catch up, or not care about that awful feeling of life passing me by. All my problems would still be there five hours later. Smoke. Repeat.

For months on this sober journey, my Higher Power revealed itself to me in the form of patience. I had to learn to sit, really sit, with my feelings, cravings, awful thoughts about myself, and life. I sit, waiting for responses instead of blowing up everything when it felt like I wasn't getting my way right away.

Today, I'm 14 months clean and sober and my life is a series of miracles. I would have never seen any of this unfolding from a process. I'm writing a show with a class that keeps me on deadline. I have the dog of my dreams; my home was given to me; my yoga students are thanking me for teaching them patience. More incredible opportunities keep coming. My family bonds are actually strengthening and I know that when something good happens to me, it is a reflection of my Higher Power's love for me.

Final thought: Today, I will surrender to the process that has worked for so many who've gone before me, to see the unique and beautiful life that is waiting for me through willingness and patience.

December 1

Carrying the Message Through Service

"We are now in a position to truly carry the message, in a powerful and joyful way, to the fellow addicts who are still suffering."

- Life with Hope, first edition, pages 63-64

I am so grateful to the fellow MA members who helped me get through the first period of recovery. I had many difficult days and there was always someone from MA who would listen to me without judgment and give me support. The kindness of MA members was an act of love. I like to give back what I first received in recovery and I am carrying the message through service. The greatest joy comes from giving and being of service. Service is a key to joy, to love.

I heard someone say, "When I got busy, I got better." Activity through service helped me in my early days of recovery. Attending a meeting, participating in a meeting, and offering help are all acts of service. When I support others, I find comfort and joy in the act of giving and being of service. The more I give to myself, the more I can give to others. I have learned to give to others from a place of inner strength and compassion. Being of service to others brings me true happiness. I realized that this loving, giving person is the real me. My true purpose in life is to give to others, and I receive happiness, fulfillment, and meaning in return. I am able to give without expecting a reward and the greatest reward is realized by helping others.

Final thought: If I want to have happiness for a lifetime, I can help somebody and be of service.

December 2

Compassion for Self and Others

"This step says that we can be of service to God, ourselves and others."

- *Life with Hope*, first edition, page 64

After coming to the program, finding a sponsor, and working the Steps, I realized that I can be of service to God, myself, and others, which is a spiritual awakening. I honor my truth, seek guidance, and serve others suffering from this disease. We would not have a fellowship if our members didn't "suit up and show up" for the necessities of Marijuana Anonymous. Through this work we engage integrity, willingness, and both compassion and self-compassion to aid others on the path of recovery. As we each develop our unique characteristics, we have, collectively, many gifts to share.

Final thought: Through giving back, we receive.

December 3

Trusting Higher Power

"If I trust the inner guidance my Higher Power gives me then I will receive all I need and more."

- Coming Home, *Life with Hope*, second edition, page 215

When I came into recovery, many years ago, fear got in the way of trusting my Higher Power. The Third Step seemed impossible to me, as I had no clue what my Higher Power was, and certainly had no trust it would be safe to turn my life over to it. At first, I had to use the group as my Higher Power and that worked well for me.

Early in my recovery, when I struggled with obsessive craving, I took the advice of a member who suggested I pray for the compulsion to use be removed. When I did, I could feel a transformation happen in the cells of my body. This really opened my eyes, that believing in a Higher Power could transform my life.

Later, after completing Steps Four through Nine, I was able to learn the limitations of my ego and its fear of letting go of control. Accepting that my ego will always be governed by fear, I needed to find another way. Developing a regular meditation practice helped to form a stronger bond with my Higher Power. I was able to feel the love, joy, and rock-solid strength of Higher Power's presence.

I began trusting this connection more and more to make decisions and lessen the fear my ego generates. This helped me change careers to one I loved, deal with the challenges of the workplace, and retire comfortably. I was able to find and marry a wonderful person and we support each other's spiritual growth. Best of all, I live a life based on trust that my Higher Power will care for me—no matter what.

Final thought: Today, I will trust the guidance of my Higher Power and will not let fear get in the way of living a life happy, joyous, and free.

December 4

Freedom to be Myself

"Marijuana gave me wings to fly, and took away the sky."

- Freedom to Be Me, *Life with Hope*, third edition, page 116

My use of marijuana spurred a progressive constriction of my freedom, potential, and connection to myself and others. As time passed during my active addiction, my dreams and ambitions were often blotted out or diminished by the smoky haze where I was existing.

It is a powerful, beautiful, and oftentimes, an intimidating realization that there is a whole world around me teeming with opportunity and possibility now that I am free of marijuana. Without marijuana, I am free in ways I never even realized; I was imprisoned.

Now I can build, enjoy, experience, and be truly present in my life. Marijuana gave me wings and took away the sky. In recovery, I am given the chance to strengthen my precious wings and a limitless sky to fly, create, and really live. With my fellows, the Steps, meetings, and my Higher Power, I can embrace my true grace, autonomy, and potential.

Final thought: Today, I acknowledge my freedom to live fully and boldly in recovery as I embrace my limitless potential.

December 5

Privately Defined World

"Some of us were delusional; we lived in a private world no one else shared."

- *Life with Hope*, first edition, page 16

My delusion seemed so very sensible in my privately-defined reality: I thought that the emptiness I felt inside would go away if I filled it up. I spent every available minute of my life stuffing whatever I could find into that hole but to my dismay, it only grew larger. I responded with "more," searching for anything to fill the void: political or religious causes, my work, creative projects, acquisitions of all kinds and, of course, lots of cannabis. The sense of emptiness only grew.

At last, I could do nothing but surrender, and I left the isolation of my addiction for the community of my fellows in recovery. I began to understand my problem in light of the word "private," from Latin, *privatus*, meaning "bereaved, deprived, separated." I came to see that what I sought came not by filling myself up with things, but rather by pouring myself into service. Empathy was reawakened in me through listening to the suffering of others and sharing in their recovery. I found satisfaction, meaning, and joy by offering my time, experience, and wisdom to others who were suffering as I had. Together, we found the fullness of communion we'd never imagined possible in our most private dreams.

Final thought: Today, I get joy by carrying the message.

December 6

Service Gives You Purpose

"Our own lives and sanity are in jeopardy if we don't help those who are still sick."

- *Life with Hope*, second edition, page 81

Early on in recovery, I remember hearing the Fifth Tradition being read at meetings. "Each group has but one primary purpose, to carry its message to the marijuana addict who still suffers." It was inspiring to think that I was part of a group that had a purpose, and not just any purpose, but a primary purpose; that purpose was to carry the message to the suffering addict. My sponsor further reinforced this mantra and the benefits of doing service, by frequently reminding me that, "service keeps you sober."

At first, I just accepted this suggestion at face value, because my early recovery was too busy for closer inspection. After many years of being clean and sober, I've gained a deeper appreciation for the many ways in which service benefits my recovery. Pausing to care about someone else's suffering gives me freedom from the bondage of ego and self-will. Putting that care into action means going to meetings, sharing my experience, making outreach calls to check on people, and even helping to organize events at district and world levels.

All these things remind me that I'm not alone, that I'm part of something larger and greater than myself. I've even modified the phrase to make it rhyme: "Service gives you purpose."

Final thought: Today, I will carry the message, not only because it helps my fellows, but also because it helps me just as much.

December 7

Progress, Not Perfection

"We strive for progress, not perfection."

- *Life with Hope*, first edition, page 33

The disease is progressive, but so is recovery. Our book says that recovery is a process, not an event. It would be simpler if there were a certificate or badge, something proving that I've arrived—that I am now sober forever. Thank you, I can now put this addiction thing behind me. It doesn't work that way and thank God it doesn't. I get to continue deepening my waters and moving in the flow of life. Every time I seek God's help, I need to knock on the door again. I must knock again to remind myself that I'm still seeking. I'm still in need.

My sobriety strengthens as I remain mindful that I am in recovery. It's never behind me; if I think that then I get ahead of myself. "More will be revealed" is one of many 12-Step sayings. I've heard plenty of old-timers say they are still surprised at how they are continuing to grow into serenity. Their relationships continue to get stronger, they are improving their abilities to forgive, and their ability to love expands beyond where it's ever been.

Final thought: Even when days are hard, I still know that as long as I stay sober, my recovery will continue to heal me in ways I cannot comprehend today.

December 8

If Sought

"Do not be discouraged; none of us are saints. Our program is not easy, but it is simple. We strive for progress, not perfection. Our experiences, before and after we entered recovery, teach us three important ideas:

- That we are marijuana addicts and cannot manage our own lives;
- That probably no human power can relieve our addiction; and
- That our Higher Power can and will if sought."

- How It Works, Life with Hope, second edition, page 227

When I first got to recovery and heard the "ABC's of the program," I realized that I have the privilege to have that gift of desperation. This meant to me that I did not know it was a problem, until it was a problem. Now, I had a choice of seeking a Higher Power. There is God's will, my will, and the choice of which to choose.

Final thought: Today, I enjoy the seeking, rather than the bag of gold.

December 9

Principles Before Personalities

"...our spiritual foundation becomes more important than our individual egos."

- Life with Hope, first edition, page 99

Whenever I am at a meeting where things get decided on a group level, I usually become more amazed at how this program must be spiritually inspired. I come together with my MA family to a safe place where we can learn and grow and let our lives become something "beyond our wildest dreams." This doesn't mean in a material sense, but by learning that I am no worse or better than anyone. I am just a druggie hoping for another 24 hours.

It took a while to believe that the people in the rooms were truly interested in my struggle. I had an experience in my early days where something I said came back to me in an uncomfortable way. At that point I had a choice; am I willing to go to any lengths and ignore this, or will I let my hurt pride take me out?

I am so glad I chose to stay and learned how important the Twelfth Tradition is, especially to vulnerable newcomers. We may grow impatient with ourselves and others. We don't get the God's eye view on anyone else's path. We can only share our own experience, strength, and hope. Gossip and grumpy comparison are human, but not helpful and can be damaging. We take our disease and recovery seriously but not ourselves. We learn to live and let live.

Final thought: Today, I know I am a child of God and a work in progress.

December 10

Service Keeps Us Clean

"As we each work the program in our own special way, we discover the spiritual principles that we all have in common. We are all unique examples of how the program works, each of us with our distinct gifts to share."

- Life with Hope, second edition, page 69

In the beginning of my recovery, I needed to take a lot. I had very little to give, but I could set up chairs or help arrange the literature at a meeting. I then mirrored what was done for me; I said hello to new faces and welcomed them to our meeting. I made and accepted program calls. When I finished my Steps, my sponsor said I could now practice Step Twelve and become a sponsor myself. The selflessness and accountability to another person required of a sponsor was a gift I never could have imagined. It is often said that a sponsor gets just as much from the sponsee as the inverse. I have been at severe lows in my recovery when a call from a sponsee picked me up and reminded me I am not alone, or distracted me from my own thoughts.

I was given lessons on how to apply the principles of recovery, traditions, and concepts of service in this work. Whether I said hello to a newcomer, served in the District, or sponsored other marijuana addicts, I have always found ways to be of service in recovery. As I find ways to share my own gifts of sobriety, my once damaged self-esteem grows and I can experience love and faith in my daily life as I never did before Marijuana Anonymous. We contribute to the legacy of this program which ensures that a strong and unified fellowship is available to the marijuana addict who still suffers and that what was given so freely to us is available for those who follow. In loving service, we recover.

Final thought: Today, with a powerful example from my sponsor, I know service keeps me clean.

December 11

Accepted and Understood

"Marijuana Anonymous is a fellowship of people who share our experience, strength and hope with each other that we may solve our common problem and help others to recover from marijuana addiction."

- Preamble, *Life with Hope*, third edition, page *xvii*

When I was using, I had withdrawn from people and became isolated; it was a very lonely feeling. I felt as though I needed to protect myself from anyone getting close to me so that I wouldn't be rejected and hurt. By coming to meetings and listening to other marijuana addicts, I did not feel so alone. I felt accepted and understood. I could learn from others who had similar problems with marijuana. I learned about recovery by listening to experiences that other people in the fellowship were having. With the support that I received, I felt strength from the fellowship. I was able to grow in my recovery. I have made many friends in recovery and enjoy the fellowship that we share.

Final thought: These days I enjoy being "happy, joyous, and free."

December 12

Turning Over My Will and My Life

"When we took this step, we were practicing the principle of faith."

- *Life with Hope*, second edition, page 11

The first time I took the Third Step, I felt the most wonderful sense of surrender. I thought I would turn over my will and my life and it would stay turned over. Well, my will is darn pesky, so I've found that I need to turn it over at least once a day, usually more often. When I worked in an office building, I trained myself to do a Third Step every time I got in an elevator, at least twice a day.

I heard in meetings that my will is my thoughts, and my life is my actions. This means I turn over my thoughts and my actions to my Higher Power, to give me good orderly direction. Over time, I've learned that I'm powerless over my first thought, but like a runaway train, I don't have to follow it. I can jump off the tracks and ask for a different thought. If need be, I call a friend in recovery to help me derail wrong thinking. By taking the Third Step, I am willing to live life a new way.

Final thought: Higher Power, help me turn to you when agitated or unsure. Give me the right thought and action.

December 13

Keep Coming Back

"Those who stop coming to meetings face a rough and lonely road."

- Life with Hope, second edition, page 74

Many in the fellowship are familiar with the phrase "Progress Not Perfection." Some of us wander off the path of recovery and can relapse back into our addiction. We have wandered away from a clearcut path that many have worked to make safe and straightforward. It leads to a destination and has fellow travelers and signs letting us know where we are heading.

The only time I stopped going to meetings was when I relapsed. I suddenly found myself in rough terrain, alone, not knowing where to turn and certainly getting cut and banged up through the metaphorical thorny bushes of my addiction. The relapse into addiction was often a direct result of feeling alone. In those moments, I was not stopping to ask fellow travelers how to keep going, I was not listening to my guide (sponsor), I stopped reading the signs and road map (The Twelve Steps). Instead, I just went my own way, giving up on the idea that anyone who'd come before me would have anything to offer.

To get lost and then come back onto the trail can feel, at first, embarrassing and full of shame. Not once did an addict on the road to recovery shame me for coming back. Instead, they held out their hand(s). Life with Hope reminds us that we do not have to face recovery alone.

Final thought: Today, I will choose to walk the path of recovery and to connect with my fellow MA addicts through a meeting, fellowship, or a phone call.

December 14

What We Could Never Do Alone

"We now have tools to help us grow. Our goals become attainable. We find ourselves in possession of new degrees of honesty, tolerance, patience, unselfishness, serenity, and love. Experience has shown us that we can all learn to live by spiritual principles"

- Life with Hope, second edition, page 63

Many people in the program have said it felt like everyone else had a manual on how to live life except for us. As an 18-year-old young man, I was confused, depressed, and unsuccessful at dealing with life on life's terms. Looking back, it's not surprising I started looking for ways to escape from my feelings. It only took a few months before I started to feel dependent on smoking weed, but it would take me years to admit that I had a problem. I was missing structure in my life, tangible goals, and people to whom I could be accountable and with whom I could be honest.

These are all things I have found in MA, and the program has given me a toolkit and a better way to live my life. The friends I've made have been on a deeper, more honest level and are working towards major goals in their lives, which motivates me. I'm trying to stay clean from marijuana, but I'm also chasing my dream job, a healthier lifestyle, and working to process old trauma. I can do this because the program is the structure I need, and the support that I was looking for but couldn't find anywhere else.

I've witnessed profound changes in other people and in myself, as I've made large strides towards my goals and engaged in the hard work required to grow. Every act of service that I've done has also been exactly the same help I needed, and so by helping others, I help myself.

Final thought: Today, doing service is an act that gives my life more purpose and meaning, and it's a way I can give back to the same pool of wisdom and serenity that I drew heavily from during my desperate early days of recovery.

December 15

Quitting the Futile Battle

"The entire foundation of our program depends on an honest admission of our powerlessness over addiction and the unmanageability of our lives."

- Life with Hope, third edition, page 5

When I reflect on the 14 years I was using, I thought I was honest with myself. I thought I could use just on the weekends, or at night, or with friends, or with whatever guardrail I chose. These efforts to control my use failed over and over and over. I wasn't purposely lying to myself. I didn't know the definition of an addict. I had never been taught the concept of powerlessness. I didn't know what I didn't know.

Fellow addicts modeled what it meant to identify powerlessness with repeated failures to control their use. I recognized the same powerlessness in my failure to control my use. Now, anytime a thought of using passes, I remember the truth. Being honest with myself, I am finally empowered to make the choice not to use. I already know where that road leads.

No matter if I'm failing in every other area, if I at least use Step One, it keeps me from using again. I'm done futilely battling with myself over trying to control my use. I'm done fighting. Quitting the battle I know I'll never win is the biggest win in itself. I'm not a fool, so I'm done fooling myself. I am an addict in recovery.

Final thought: Today, I choose to surrender my former, ignorant self to my future, wise self.

December 16

We Carry Each Other

"Some of the greatest pleasure and privilege in service comes from sponsorship."

- Life with Hope, first edition, page 65

I had tried for many years to control my using. I could control my using for periods of time but eventually I would find myself back into that terrible cycle. When I approached my sponsor, I felt that if I wanted this to work, I had to be honest with her. She was hard-core, old-school and it was exactly what I needed. I had been lying for so long that even I believed my stories and excuses. I had a hard time trusting people but for some reason I trusted her.

She taught me to be on time and do what I said I was going to do. She showed me that this was an illness; not a "good person/bad person" thing. She told me that my feelings would not kill me but my actions were what counted. She let me know that esteemable acts brought about self-esteem. She acknowledged there was a lot of unfairness in the world but seeing myself as a victim would not serve me nor my spiritual growth. After a while, I learned to listen without judgment in the meetings and also to listen to what I was telling myself.

I have had the privilege of sponsoring many women and some stayed, some returned, some became like a healthy family. We laugh at things that normal folks might find appalling. We carry each other through tough times by knowing that we are truly lucky to have left our old ways behind; one day at a time.

Final thought: Today, I support my program by staying in close contact with others who have recovery as their primary purpose.

December 17

It Works

"I will always remember my first Marijuana Anonymous meeting. I was scared and nervous, but I remember all of that melting away as the meeting started. Soon I realized, 'this is where I need to be.'"

- *Sharing Our Experience, Strength, and Hope, Personal Stories of Marijuana Addicts,*
MA pamphlet

I remember my first MA meeting; I was in a very confused and depressed place. I couldn't imagine how to let go of marijuana, but I knew I had to if I wanted to have a better life. I had just had a brief stay in a psych ward and I recognized even then that marijuana heavily contributed to that bottom. When I entered the meeting, I felt welcomed and comfortable. My thoughts were like a tornado, but the people there had a calmness that helped me stay through the meeting. I heard the Steps for the first time. They were daunting, overwhelming, and filled with the promise of hard work but also reward. I wanted to be on the other side of the Steps, living a better life but I didn't know how to get there or if I actually could.

The people at the meeting stood out to me. Their recovery and wisdom were powerful and tangible. I was in a great fog and seemingly stuck in my ways, but I still noticed how positively they talked of change and overcoming life's hard times. They were free, confident, relaxed, and grounded; I wanted that too. I had a few good conversations in that room, and I left feeling more worthy and capable of making the changes needed. I was doubtful, but I kept coming back and I started to see real benefits in my life from MA meetings and working the Steps.

Final thought: Today, I have the opportunity to pay it forward and help newcomers feel safe, too. I can share some of my hope, strength, and experience and do service. Any marijuana addict can also have serenity in their lives one day at a time, thanks to MA.

December 18

Time is Not a Tool

"Continuous and thorough action is essential to our recovery."

- Life with Hope, second edition, page 68

After many years in Marijuana Anonymous, I know that if my brain was to tell me I'm not an addict and maybe I can use again, it's my addiction talking. Gratefully, I've never lost my fear of going back to being a slave to marijuana. It quit working long before I was able to quit. I have a daily reprieve IF I continue to attend meetings, work the Steps with a sponsor, and give away what I have been so freely given.

Early on, I heard a member say, "Time is not a tool." This tells me that no matter how long I've been clean, my years don't keep me clean today. Time shows me that I can get through all kinds of experiences staying clean but I still need to do the work.

When I was new, I thought the tools would be different when I had more time; but I've discovered that the tools are always the same, no matter whether I have a day or 10 years: going to meetings, working the steps, and working with others.

Final thought: I wake up each morning and give thanks for another day, and ask to stay clean for this 24 hours.

December 19

Ego Deflation

"Here is where I realized what this program is really about - the deflation of my ego. The program taught me that humility is the solution and learning to be humble was the answer to my ego problem."

-My Best Thinking Got Me Here, *Life with Hope*, second edition, page 177

I was full of myself when I came into Marijuana Anonymous. I was self-centered and incapable of seeing the world through anyone else's perspective but my own. My ego was my own worst enemy. I was always worried that I wouldn't get what I wanted and I lived in perpetual fear. When I came to my first MA meeting there wasn't really any other place for me to go. I had burned many bridges and had few friends who wanted me around.

I was amazed at what I heard and for the first time in a long time felt like I belonged somewhere. As I got into recovery I was asked to do service, set up chairs, greet people at the door, and then chair meetings and take on service commitments. As I worked these Steps I learned new principles that allowed me to overcome my fear and ego and to start seeing the world through a new set of eyes. I learned that it wasn't all about me. The more I put the thoughts of others in front of my own, the more my world opened. I understood that humility is the true goal of this program.

Final thought: Today, I will let go of what I want and work on how I can be of service to others.

December 20

We Recover Together

"We take these steps for ourselves, not by ourselves. Others have gone before; others will follow. We recover."

- Life with Hope, second edition, page 69

Before finding recovery, I thought asking for help was a sign of weakness. I struggled for years trying to quit smoking pot on a daily basis. I didn't know there was a different way to live, and that with recovery tools, I could lose the obsession and compulsion to use a drug that no longer served me. I heard in a meeting that when we start with pot, it's magic, then it becomes medicine and in the end, it's only misery. This was definitely my experience. I used pot long after it was fun or enjoyable. When I finally was told about recovery and went to a meeting, I remember feeling bewildered and unsure what to do, but at least I wasn't using.

Once the fog of smoke lifted, I understood that while I couldn't quit on my own, alone, I could quit with the help of other addicts. It took me a few months to have the courage to ask someone to be my sponsor and to help me work these Steps. Nothing has ever made lasting changes as much as these Twelve Steps. The steps are real magic! I'm grateful I learned that it takes strength to ask for help; that it's not a sign of weakness. I don't have to do this recovery alone. Any time that I can pick up that 500 lb. phone, I can reach out to a fellow addict and get the support I need. There is a fellowship and it supports each and every one of us.

Final thought: Today, I know I am part of a worldwide fellowship of marijuana addicts that help each other stay clean, one day at a time.

December 21

Sincerely Unique

"We are all unique examples of how the program works, each of us with our distinct gifts to share."

- *Life with Hope*, second edition, page 69

In recovery, I've learned there's no such thing as being "terminally unique." To me, the phrase means that no one's character or circumstances are so unique that the only path forward is utter despair or death. I've heard enough grumbling from newcomers to think this phrase can sometimes turn them off. They walk away with the impression, "These recovery people think everyone is the same, and no one is special." I really appreciate that Marijuana Anonymous has a culture of appreciating that each one of us is unique.

This is a program with a solution for people with the shared condition of being marijuana addicts but it doesn't ask us to shed what makes us special. Through working the Twelve Steps of MA and participating in the fellowship, I've been able to bring all of my special qualities to the surface and finally begin to reach my potential.

Final thought: Today, I will sincerely share my distinct gifts with the world and help others find their ability to do so.

December 22

Strength Through Spiritual Growth

"As we make spiritual progress, we begin to feel emotionally secure. Our new attitudes bring about self-esteem, inner strength, and serenity that is not easily shaken by any of life's hard times."

- Life with Hope, second edition, page 68

Whether completely sober or in active drug use, life will always bring about adversity, because challenging times are inevitable. Life never gets easier—we just get stronger, but only when we work a spiritual program as addicts in recovery. In Marijuana Anonymous, I continue to grow spiritually; I cultivate areas of my life that I once had little to no agency over (despite these areas being things I can control), including my self-esteem, inner strength, and serenity. In essence, I'm in control of my emotional sobriety, and spiritual progress is the vessel that propels me forward into a life full of resilience. I no longer cower when I'm in the presence of fear, but rather, I lean into my faith through the spiritual muscles I continually grow each day. Through my spiritual awakening, as a result of the 12 Steps of Marijuana Anonymous, I have the freedom to live a meaningful life—so long as I continue to practice the principles in all of my affairs.

Final thought: Today, I choose to practice the principles of this spiritual program so that my faith will continue to strengthen and carry me through any challenging circumstance that stands in my way.

December 23

Our Primary Purpose

"The existence of MA depends on the preservation of Tradition Five"

- Life with Hope, second edition, page 81

Our primary purpose is to carry our message to the marijuana addict who still suffers. Our message is one of hope, that anyone can recover from marijuana addiction with the support of other addicts in Marijuana Anonymous. Before I came into recovery, I had no idea how meetings were going to help me. I only knew that I was sick and tired of marijuana and I could not quit on my own, no matter how hard I tried.

It was at my second meeting that I realized everyone in the room was relying on everyone else in the room to help them stay clean, one day at a time. I left that second meeting with the thought in my head that I only had to quit smoking pot one day at a time.

I made it through the next day without smoking pot, which was a miracle and then I made it another day. During that first week I sometimes went one hour at a time. I heard stories of people who relapsed because they had stopped going to meetings, which encouraged me to continue going to meetings no matter what. I lost the obsession and compulsion right away, for which I'm grateful. I welcome newcomers like I was welcomed. When I share my story of how I came into MA with a newcomer, I remember what it was like, and how much I've learned since that first day.

Final thought: Today, I am willing to be of service to the addict who is still suffering.

December 24

Higher Powered

"We can stop and ask God for guidance. Our Higher Power's guidance will let us use our great human faculty, our intuition. We can live life with some wisdom and a great deal of wit. We gain more trust in God, ourselves, and other human beings."

- Life with Hope, first edition, page 53

After choosing to embrace and believe in a Higher Power, I no longer need to live in doubt and fear. Instead, I am able to live in a space where my intuition, through God's guidance, will ultimately lead to the next indicated right step of action. By no longer relying on my own self-will, my Higher Power's will for me can make every situation acceptable, knowing my Higher Power is in control. I can live with my faith that everything happens for a reason under God's eyes; thus, I can trust the process of life, including myself, and those around me.

Final thought: Today, I am able to act according to any situation, because I have the moral guidance from my Higher Power.

December 25

Giving to Receive

"This Step says we can be of service to God, ourselves, and others. Those of us that have been around long enough to take all the Steps are well aware that this kind of giving is its own reward. The more we help others, the more we help ourselves."

- Life with Hope, second edition, page 64

Throughout my time in recovery and after working the Steps, I found a purpose in life, finding a lot of direction from the Saint Francis/ Eleventh Step Prayer and from being of service. While others may see what's lacking, I task myself to see what I can bring to the table and fill that hole. It can be carrying the message in any way that I can or embracing who I truly am and living authentically to show others that there's a place in the world and in the rooms for them, too.

One of the greatest gifts that I've gotten from MA and one that I've had the opportunity to continue to give away over and over again, is the power of fellowship. I'm fortunate that my home group is on Friday night in Los Angeles. After each meeting we go out for fellowship, sharing a meal and having some laughs, staying out super late, like we're not missing out on anything in life being clean. Our literature says sharing good times with fellow addicts lets newcomers see that it is possible to enjoy life in recovery.

When I first realized that there was fun to be had in sobriety, the possibilities seemed endless and that was when my life with hope began. In helping to continue the tradition of fellowship and bringing joy, laughter and fun into other people's lives, the love I give, in return, fills up my own cup. Things fall into place and everything in my life seems right where it's supposed to be.

Final thought: Today, I will be of service to my fellows and the people around me–bringing some light, love, and laughter into the world.

December 26

The Gifts of Recovery

"As we move away from the chaos of our former lives, we begin to truly experience peace and serenity. We now find ourselves in a new state of mind where we can strengthen our relationship with a loving God."

- Life with Hope, second edition, page 53

While life without weed is on the whole so much better than when I was using every day, there are still times when my addict mind tells me I'm missing out. I find myself wishing I could just smoke a joint or drink a beer like a "normal person." When this happens, I've found it helpful to get myself to a meeting and to remember all I've gained in recovery, rather than what I've lost.

I remember that I'm grateful for:

A clear conscience,

Less anxiety and paranoia,

Being able to look neighbors in the eye,

A clearer, less foggy mind.

A healthier body and

The confidence my Higher Power is present in my life.

Final thought: Acknowledging these gifts of recovery brings me peace and reminds me that I wouldn't trade them for any amount of weed in my life.

December 27

Recovery in Action

"Continuous and thorough action is essential to our recovery."

- Life with Hope, second edition, page 68

I've heard the phrase "talk is cheap," but in this program, I began acting on it for the first time in my life. Certainly, there's nothing wrong with having good intentions and saying kind words to those around us; however, intentions and words are minor factors in comparison with the power of action. When I do my Fourth Step, I am reminded that it is a writing exercise, not a thinking exercise. Writing is the action I use to clear out old blockages and release emotions and energies that have been pent up for many years.

When I do my Ninth Step, I take action in the form of amending my behavior, changing the patterns of harm that I've neglected for all my life. I make meaningful amends to those I harmed, while making sure not to exacerbate that harm to them or others.

When I do my Twelfth Step, I remember that faith without works is dead. I take action in the form of giving service at meetings, helping to plan and organize recovery events, and sponsoring newcomers to facilitate their Step work. Even a five-minute phone call can be a powerful and life-altering action, if I use it to connect with another living soul. This is a spiritual program, but it is also a program of action. The spiritual life is not a theory; I must live it. I do not need to arrive at perfection, but I do need to put my principles into practice through action.

Final thought: Today, let me remember that recovery is not an event. It's a process, and it requires action!

December 28

Imagining Higher Power

"I first imagined my Higher Power to be two oak trees holding up a hammock. I would lie in the hammock being held. Finally I gave up trying to figure out my Higher Power."

- A Slave To Marijuana, Life with Hope, second edition, page 119

During my using, I spent so much time trying to precisely identify what I believed about spirituality. I found a concept of a Higher Power that I could show off to my friends while we passed a blunt around. When the party was over, I put my Higher Power back in the box and up on the shelf. It had no impact on my daily life.

When I got clean, I needed to find a Higher Power that could work in my life to restore me to sanity. I started praying by listening to music with intention. "This minimum of belief is enough to open the door and cross the threshold" (Life with Hope, first edition, page 7). During my sobriety, my Higher Power has been many different things. Just as my recovery grows and develops every day, so too does my relationship with my Higher Power. Where I start doesn't matter, as long as I do in fact start.

Final thought: Today, I embrace my relationship with my Higher Power, as I understand my Higher Power, in this moment.

December 29

Pull for Shore!

"We take these steps for ourselves, not by ourselves...we recover."

- Life with Hope, second edition, page 69

My addiction story is one of complete isolation. I had decided the solution to my issues and complaints was to never come down. I sat alone, ate Doritos and cried. A friend said, "Get out of the house, even if you have to tell yourself 'no one will throw rocks at me.' " Those first steps took me to a meeting. There I found friends willing to pull me into that lifeboat, and show me how to row for the shore.

Today, I live in gratitude, helping my newest friends into the grace of a life worth living; into the lifeboat. I am not alone anymore. I have sponsors, sponsees, fellow addicts and friends, and a Higher Power I heard someone call "Poppa." My minimal desire was to just find sanity but it took Step Twelve to really accept the blossoming of a spiritual connection. Now, I feel that connection in everything I do. I found a way out of the toxic atmosphere and into the light. I share that light in everything I do. My new life is a blessing, achieved through prayer, meditation, and going to phone and land meetings, and no one throws rocks at me.

Final thought: Today, I live in gratitude, helping my newest friends into the grace of a life worth living; into the lifeboat.

December 30

Being of Service

"Service work provides the backbone of our MA; if there is no service, there is no program... It is our responsibility to do what we can to make sure that MA continues to be there for us, for the marijuana addict who still suffers, and for the addict who is not yet born."

- Life with Hope, second edition, page 65

It is said in the rooms over and over that service will keep me clean, but I think people miss that service also keeps Marijuana Anonymous alive. From starting new meetings to attending a meeting and not saying a word, every act of service gives my program of recovery a day more of life. In turn, it gives life back to the addict who is still suffering, close to spiritual death. It is through my continuous dedication to recovery that I show others the gifts I receive, and it is through service that I give back what was so freely given.

There is a unique feeling of completion that comes with helping another addict. Service can also occur at work, church, school, the grocery store, in my home with my family, and on the phone with customer service. There are countless opportunities to spread a message of hope by simply giving freely. When in doubt, imagine a world in which no one took the time to be of service to others. Remember that every day, our work inside and outside of the rooms makes a difference.

Final thought: Today, I will find a way to be of service. It helps me stay clean, helps others, and keeps the world turning, no matter what room I'm in.

December 31

Being of Service for Myself

"The greatest satisfaction of recovery and living life by the spiritual principles of the Twelve Steps comes when we give it away."

- Life with Hope, second edition, page 64

The most important thing that I can do according to Step Twelve, is to give it away and be of service to MA—the fellowship that saved my life. I show my gratitude, and ensure MA continues to exist for my fellow addicts, by being of service. Step Twelve explains that "our survival depends upon a healthy and functioning fellowship. It is our responsibility to do what we can to make sure that MA continues to be there." If we fail to give back, MA would cease to exist.

When I once thanked my sponsor, she said I could thank her by sponsoring others. In doing so, I am able to get out of my own cluttered, anxiety-ridden, and self-involved mind, and in turn think about others. I can also be of service by being a reader or timer in a meeting, a secretary, or serving at the District-level or on World Services' Committee. We can even be of service just by attending a meeting. Someone with one month can even offer reassurance to a newcomer at their first meeting. All of these ways of being of service are vital to MA's existence.

Service strengthens my recovery, my relationships with others, and my self-esteem. Some of the greatest moments of joy come from my developed ability to help others. It gives me a sense of purpose I lacked before when I was in active addiction. As it says in Step Twelve, which is true in my own life "the more we help others, the more we help ourselves." Through practicing the principles and being of service, I have been "transformed from [a] suffering addict" into someone who is "happy, joyous, and free."

Final thought: As another year ends and a new one begins, I resolve to find ways to be of service, and give away what was so freely given to me so MA can continue to exist for myself, my fellows, the marijuana addict who still suffers, and the addict who is yet to be born.

Index

Fear: January 1, 11, 26, 31; February 6, 8, 9, 13, 18, 23, 29; March 5, 6, 14, 16, 23, 26, 28, 29; April 7, 14, 15, 16, 22, 30; May 2, 3, 7, 10, 13, 14, 16, 23, 26, 28, 30; June 4, 7, 23, 26, 29; July 5, 10, 11, 15, 16, 18, 20, 24, 28; August 17, 19, 29; September 10, 19, 25, 30; October 3, 5, 15; November 1, 4, 14; December 3, 18, 19, 22, 24

Fearless Moral Inventory: February 8; October 3

Feelings: January 16, 21, 23, 26; February 10, 11; March 3, 12, 16, 23, 28; April 1, 8, 15, 24; May 16, 22, 26, 30; June 4, 6, 9, 10, 13, 20, 25; July 6, 11, 28; August 6, 12, 26, 27, 29; September 18, 25, 26; October 5, 11, 21, 25, 27; November 4, 15, 16, 30; December 14, 16

Fellowship: January 2, 16, 31; February 2, 6, 18, 21; March 7; April 2, 4, 11, 17, 18, 23, 27, 28; May 5, 6, 21, 22, 28, 29; June 6, 10, 14, 23, 25, 27; July 5, 12, 13, 14, 16, 21, 24, 27; August 3, 8, 9, 14, 18, 20, 30; September 6, 8, 10, 12, 27, 28; October 15, 17, 24, 31; November 1, 5, 18, 19, 21, 29; December 2, 10, 11, 13, 20, 21, 25, 31

Forgiveness: January 25; March 3; April 9, 30; June 1; September 1, 9; October 1, 11, 15; November 5

Freedom: January 1, 2, 13, 23, 31; February 16, 22, 29; March 11, 27; April 13, 25, 28, 29; May 4, 23, 29; June 7, 8; July 3, 10, 14, 16, 18, 21, 29; August 10, 12, 13, 17, 25, 28, 31; September 6, 27; November 15; December 4, 6, 22

God of My Understanding: February 11, 14, 19, 25; March 1, 11; June 7; July 17, 31; August 21, 23; September 5, 8; October 7, 9, 12, 16; November 6

Grace: February 8, 12; March 22, April 19; June 8, 15, 22; July 9, 14; August 7; September 6, 8, 10, 21, 23, 28, 29; October 6; November 12; December 4, 29

Grateful: January 14, 28, 30; February 1, 3, 9, 13, 18, 19, 23, 24; March 4, 6, 14, 29; April 1, 6, 16, 18, 28; May 16; June 6, 30; July 4, 6, 10, 12, 15, 16, 21, 24, 30; August 7, 9, 17, 18, 19, 28; September 3, 6, 8, 14, 27, 29; October 6, 7, 10, 13, 17, 24, 25; November 1, 2, 4, 5, 9, 12, 13, 21; December 1, 18, 20, 23, 26

Gratitude: January 21, 27, 30; March 7, 29; April 2; May 16, 25; June 11, 13, 28, 30; July 18, 19, 28; August 5, 19; September 1, 9, 11, 14, 29; October 15, 24; November 5, 11, 13, 28; December 29

Guilt: January 21, 25, 26; February 9; March 3, 6, 13; April 8; May 7, 9; July 7, 18; August 28; September 25

Honesty: January 2, 5, 8, 17, 28; March 16; April 2, 8, 10, 11, 19, 30; May 5, 9, 26; June 18; July 7; August 4, 12, 16, 25; October 3, 13, 15; November 3, 17; December 14

Hope: January 11, 31; February 4; March 18; April 2, 11, 28, 30; May 3, 10, 18, 21, 28; July 3, 14; August 5, 9, 10, 11; September 5-7, 9, 11, 15, 22; October 11, 15, 23; November 7, 17, 22; December 25, 30

Hopeless(ness): January 1, 3; February 18; March 22; April 26, 28; May 3; June 29; July 19; August 10, 11, 19, 25, 28; September 4, 12; October 5

Humility: January 4, 11, 12; February 13, 17; March 16, 19, 30; April 16, 23, 30; May 5, 9, 16; June 5, 11, 17, 30; July 7, 8, 13, 14, 19, 25; August 17, 25; September 5, 6, 10, 11, 19, 23; October 4, 15; November 3, 17, 27; December 19

Integrity: January 11, 29; February 8; March 13; May 14, 22; July 17; September 6, 7; October 8; November 3, 17; December 2

Insanity: January 31; February 8, 22; April 1, 7, 15, 30; May 3, 7, 9, 14; June 7, 28, 29; July 18, 24; September 13, 30; October 1, 3, 4, 12; November 21, 26

Isolation: January 28; February 4, 12; March 10; April 8; May 2, 18, 30; June 6; August 1, 4; September 26; October 13; December 5, 29

Loneliness: February 4, 11; March 13; April 8; May 23, 30; July 16; September 12

Meditation: January 27, 28; February 14; March 12, 19, 21; April 8, 19; June 13, 21; July 11, 18, 22, 25, 27; August 2, 21; September 9, 25; October 21; November 2, 4, 5, 10, 12, 14, 15, 23, 25, 26, 29; December 3, 29

Newcomer(s): January 16; April 2; May 5, 6, 22; June 25; July 2, 4; August 3, 9; September 10; October 3, 20, 23, 26, 31; November 6, 19; December 9, 10, 17, 21, 23, 25, 27, 31

Open-minded(ness): March 18; June 12; August 4, 18; September 9; November 3

Openness: April 20; May 9; August 12, 26; October 25; November 3

Paranoia: January 1; March 10; April 10; May 17, 28; December 26

Peace: January 1, 13, 29; February 4, 15, 16, 18; March 2, 4, 6, 12, 29; April 25, 29; May 1, 16, 26; June 2, 11, 13; July 14, 16, 25, 28; August 1; September 4, 9, 24; October 27; November 5, 11, 15, 24, 25, 28; December 26

Perfection(ism): February 14, 28; March 28; April 17; July 15; September 1; October 1, 17; November 24; December 27

Powerless(ness): January 1, 5, 8, 13, 15, 17, 19; February 1, 4; March 11, 15, 17, 18, 22; April 5, 7, 26; May 11, 13, 24, 31; June 2, 11, 16, 24; July 19, 21, 29; August 1, 18, 25, 31; September 3, 4, 19, 27; October 17, 22, 28; November 7, 9, 22, 24; December 12, 15

Prayer: January 28; February 14; March 1, 4, 12, 16, 25; April 8, 9, 11, 12, 19, 30; May 1, 26; June 21; July 17, 18, 25, 27; August 2, 10, 21, 23; September 2, 9, 25; October 21; November 2, 5, 8, 10, 12, 23, 26, 28, 29; December 25, 29

> **Serenity Prayer**: January 12; April 12; May 26; September 2; November 1, 8

> **Seventh Step Prayer**: November 8

> **Third Step Prayer**: March 4, 16, 25; November 8

Primary Purpose: May 6, 22; August 25; October 23; November 19; December 6, 16, 23

Progress: January 12; April 24; July 18; June 17; August 30; September 10; October 1, 13, 17, 26; December 9, 22; *also see Slogans, "Progress Not Perfection"*

Promises: January 25; May 16; August 4; September 11, 28; October 5

Relapse: January 25, 26, 28; February 12, 20, 21; March 7; April 8 May 15, 30; June 1, 21, 22; August 15; November 4; December 13, 23

Resentment(s): April 1, 5, 7, 13, 14, 15, 29; May 3, 7, 9, 13-16; June 1, 15; July 18; August 4, 14; September 13, 21, 29, 30; October 5, 11; November 277

Self-Acceptance: January 9; June 15; July 28

Self-Esteem: February 2, 13, 15; March 10, 11, 14, 29; April 8; May 20; June 15; July 15; August 17; October 27; December 10, 16, 22, 31

Self-Pity: January 21; March 19; July 26; August 19; September 21; October 4

Self-Respect: January 3; June 25; July 15

Self-Will: March 4, 8, 11, 15, 25, 31; May 10, 19, 20; June 3, 9; July 20, 25, 31; August 17; October 29; November 4, 5, 16, 17; December 6, 24

Serenity: January 1, 4, 30; February 15, 16, 18; March 10, 12, 16, 24, 29; April 3, 4, 8, 14, 22, 25, 29; May 4, 15, 18-20, 26, 28; June 2, 7, 13, 18, 24; July 5, 8, 16, 19, 25, 28; August 5, 10, 21, 23, 25; September 5, 23; October 13, 27; November 5, 14, 17, 23, 25; December 7, 14, 17, 22, 26

Service: January 5, 17, 26; February 12, 18, 21, 24, 29; March 13, 16, 21, 29; April 4; May 3, 8, 11, 12, 14, 18, 22, 26; June 3, 6, 11, 25, 26, 30; July 2, 4, 5, 14, 24, 27, 29; August 3, 9, 25; September 4, 9, 11, 30; October 13, 15, 17, 24; November 5, 17, 19, 26; December 1, 2, 5, 6, 10, 14, 16, 17, 19, 23, 25, 27, 30, 31

Shame: January 1, 21, 25, 31; February 1, 8, 9; March 6, 13; April 8, 10, 16, 22; May 7, 9, 27; July 18, 28; August 12, 21, 28; September 5, 25; December 13

Shortcomings: May 5; July 9, 13, 14; September 9

Slogans:

    "Easy Does It": April 2; May 20

    "Happy, Joyous, and Free": January 22; February 16, 18; March 24; April 25; May 1, 16; June 8; July 16; August 6, 20; November 9; December 3, 11, 31

    "Let Go & Let God": January 22; February 15, 23; March 22; April 22; May 12, 20; June 13; July 22; August 5; September 24; October 2, 12; November 4, 14

    "One Day at a Time": January 1; February 16, 26; March 7, 27, 28; April 10, 20, 25; May 7, 11, 19, 20, 21, 26, 29, 30; June 25, 28; July 24; August 1, 5, 7, 10, 20, 25; September 15, 29; October 10, 13, 18, 27, 29; December 16, 17, 20, 23

    "Progress Not Perfection": January 1, 22; February 28; March 28; April 19, 22; May 6; June 15; July 1, 12, 15; August 8; October 17, 26; December 7, 8, 13

372

Step Eleven: January 22, 27; March 9, 16; June 14; July 22, 28; August 21; November 8, 10, 23, 27; December 25; *also see Conscious Contact, Meditation, Prayer*

Step Twelve: March 16; December 10, 27, 29, 31; *also see Service, Sponsor, Sponsorship*

Surrender: January 22, 23, 26; February 1, 5; March 5; April 4, 16; May 15, 28, 31; June 2, 11, 16, 24; July 12, 19, 29, 31; August 1, 11; September 19, 21, 28; October 2, 9, 18; November 8, 9, 20, 24, 30; December 5, 12, 15

Turn(ing) It Over: March 11, 15, 22; April 9; May 14; June 24; July 10; September 30; October 2; December 12

Twelve Questions: January 6; February 1, 7; April 10; June 25; September 18

Tradition(s): May 6, 22; September 15; October 6, 20, 31; November 19; December 6, 9, 10, 23, 25

Unity: February 21; April 2; September 10; October 6, 31; November 10

Willing(ness): January 11, 13, 14, 18, 24, 28; February 3, 24, 27; March 2, 5, 7, 11, 19, 30; April 3, 10, 13, 20, 30; May 7, 14, 15, 25, 26, 30; June 1, 5, 7, 9, 11, 15, 26, 28; July 5, 14, 23-25; August 3, 4, 12, 18, 25, 28, 30; September 6, 7, 10, 13, 19, 22, 27; October 3, 15, 17, 21, 29; November 3, 17, 30; December 2, 9, 12, 23, 29

How It Works

The practice of rigorous honesty, of opening our hearts and minds, and the willingness to go to any lengths to have a spiritual awakening are essential to our recovery.

Our old ideas and ways of life no longer work for us. Our suffering shows us that we need to let go absolutely. We surrender ourselves to a Power greater than ourselves.

Here are the steps we take which are suggested for recovery:

1. We admitted we were powerless over marijuana, that our lives had become unmanageable.

2. Came to believe that a power greater than ourselves could restore us to sanity.

3. Made a decision to turn our will and our lives over to the care of God, as we understood God.

4. Made a searching and fearless moral inventory of ourselves.

5. Admitted to God, to ourselves, and to another human being the exact nature of our wrongs.

6. Were entirely ready to have God remove all these defects of character.

7. Humbly asked God to remove our shortcomings.

8. Made a list of all persons we had harmed, and became willing to make amends to them all.

9. Made direct amends to such people wherever possible, except when to do so would injure them or others.

10. Continued to take personal inventory and when we were wrong, promptly admitted it.

11. Sought through prayer and meditation to improve our conscious contact with God, as we understood God, praying only for knowledge of God's will for us and the power to carry that out.

12. Having had a spiritual awakening as the result of these steps, we tried to carry this message to marijuana addicts and to practice these principles in all our affairs.

Do not be discouraged, none of us are saints. Our program is not easy, but it is simple. We strive for progress, not perfection. Our experiences, before and after we entered recovery, teach us three important ideas:

- that we are marijuana addicts and cannot manage our own lives;
- that probably no human power can relieve our addiction; and
- that our Higher Power can and will, if sought.

374

The Twelve Traditions of Marijuana Anonymous

1. Our common welfare should come first; personal recovery depends upon MA unity.

2. For our group purpose there is but one ultimate authority, a loving God whose expression may come through in our group conscience. Our leaders are but trusted servants; they do not govern.

3. The only requirement for membership is a desire to stop using marijuana.

4. Each group should be autonomous except in matters affecting other groups or MA as a whole.

5. Each group has but one primary purpose, to carry its message to the marijuana addict who still suffers.

6. MA groups ought never endorse, finance, or lend the MA name to any related facility or outside enterprise, lest problems of money, property, and prestige divert us from our primary purpose.

7. Every MA group ought to be fully self-supporting, declining outside contributions.

8. Marijuana Anonymous should remain forever nonprofessional, but our service centers may employ special workers.

9. MA, as such, ought never be organized, but we may create service boards or committees directly responsible to those they serve.

10. Marijuana Anonymous has no opinion on outside issues; hence the MA name ought never be drawn into public controversy.

11. Our public relations policy is based on attraction rather than promotion; we need always maintain personal anonymity at the level of press, radio, TV, film, and other public media. We need guard with special care the anonymity of all fellow MA members.

12. Anonymity is the spiritual foundation of all our traditions, ever reminding us to place principles before personalities.

The Twelve Questions of Marijuana Anonymous

The following questions may help you determine whether marijuana is a problem in your life.

1. Has using marijuana stopped being fun?

2. Do you ever get high alone?

3. Is it hard for you to imagine a life without marijuana?

4. Do you find that your friends are determined by your marijuana use?

5. Do you use marijuana to avoid dealing with your problems or to cope with your feelings?

6. Has your marijuana use led to financial difficulties and/or legal consequences?

7. Does your marijuana use let you live in a privately defined world?

8. Have you ever failed to keep promises you made about cutting down or controlling your use of marijuana?

9. Has your use of marijuana caused problems with your health, memory, concentration, or motivation?

10. When your stash is nearly empty, do you feel anxious or worried about how to get more?

11. Do you plan your life around your marijuana use?

12. Have friends or relatives ever complained that your using is damaging your relationship with them?

If you answered yes to any of the above questions, you may have a problem with marijuana.

Updated by the 2021 MA World Service Conference, May 31, 2021

The Twelve Step Spiritual Principles

Step One: Honesty

Step Two: Hope

Step Three: Faith

Step Four: Courage

Step Five: Integrity

Step Six: Willingness

Step Seven: Humility

Step Eight: Reflection

Step Nine: Justice

Step Ten: Perseverance

Step Eleven: Spiritual Awareness

Step Twelve: Service

Resources

Find meetings, various resources, and contribute online at: Marijuana-Anonymous.org.

Download the Marijuana Anonymous app for your mobile device. Find these resources and more on the app:

Life with Hope, second edition

Life with Hope 12 Step Workbook

MA Pamphlets

Sobriety Date Counter

Meeting Finder

www.ingramcontent.com/pod-product-compliance
Lightning Source LLC
Chambersburg PA
CBHW060757120626
46557CB00001B/11